Practical Massage for Home Use

By Rafael Benjamin L.M.T.

ISBN: 0615640281

ISBN-13: 9780615640280

LCCN: 2012939288

CreateSpace, North Charleston, SC

Disclaimer: Massage should be given to healthy individuals. If a person suffers from disease that can be spread through blood stimulation, it would be advisable to get a doctor's approval first.

Table of Contents

Chapter - 3
Massage – Facing Down

Chapter - 4
Finishing Touches

Opening Remarks

It has been said that "the best things in life are free". Giving a massage to your loved one or receiving a massage, can be one of those free best things. Massage can help you bond with your mate and make you feel so wonderful. Receiving a good massage is one of the greatest pleasures in life. If you haven't tried it, you have no idea what you have been missing. It's truly a great treat, as most of you already know.

Giving a massage should not scare you either. All you really need is the desire to give of yourself to your loved one and a little know-how that this book will provide.

The following are practical massage techniques that the layperson can easily use in the comfort and the privacy of his home. It has been beautifully illustrated, and the movements are explained step by step in simple, everyday language.

Your mate, family member, or friend will greatly appreciate your massage. It will demonstrate your caring and affection to that person. When giving a massage you are taking the time and focusing your full attention on somebody else.

Giving a massage can be a very intimate activity. Let's face it, massage involves lots of touching, rubbing and pressing. All the strokes are done by hands on a body usually other than yourself. No wonder massage has been recommended for couples as a great activity to do for each other. I hope that by practicing these techniques, you will receive enjoyment from both being the receiver and the giver of massage.

Foreword

Once in a while, a book comes along that accomplishes all that it is intended to achieve. This book successfully communicates a greater understanding of the usefulness and techniques of massage. This book makes its debut during a period when holistic healing practices are becoming more and more integrated into the health-care forefront.

Individuals are being urged to take charge of their own health, to become more acquainted with how their body functions, and to trust in the healing powers of the body's innate intelligence.

The timing of a book of this nature is perfect for anyone seeking the personal fulfillment of a new heightened awareness of the therapeutic benefits of massage.

It has been my great pleasure to work with Mr. Rafael Benjamin. His gift of caring for others, of giving for the sake of giving, and his enthusiasm for life is reflected in the spirit of his fine book.

Robert Benevento, D.C.

About the Author

My name is Rafael Benjamin. I am a professional massage therapist. I must have given thousands of massages through the years. This is one of very few books that I know about that is written with the common person in mind. This book describes a complete full-body massage, literally from head to toe. At one time massage was only for wealthy individuals who could afford it. Today, however, it is becoming more and more available almost to everyone. Some medical insurance companies have taken notice of the public needs for massage and have started covering it in their plans. Massage is becoming popular among young and old alike. In spite of that, many individuals who really need a massage have not received one yet. Some may not have the money to go to a massage therapist and some may have reservations about revealing themselves in front of a stranger. This book is dedicated to those who have partners and who would like to share that experience with them but don't know how to go about it yet. Massage is hard to do on yourself, but still possible. Usually there is a giver and a receiver. In some ways receiving a massage is like receiving a kiss. In order to enjoy it, you have to share it.

My passion for massage started at a young age. When I was in elementary school, we used to have a neighbor who suffered badly from lower back pain. She asked me several times if I wouldn't mind walking on her back. I was very shy, so I said no. That went on for a while. Every time she saw me, she used to ask for my help. One day out of curiosity, I said "yes". She was very pleased. We went to her home and from there to her bedroom. She lay down on her stomach right there on the cold floor. She told me to take off my shoes and climb on top of her back. She directed my feet to her butt and asked me to walk very slowly toward her upper back. I remember trying to keep my balance. I was afraid I might fall on top of her. When I finally walked all the way to her shoulders, she asked me to walk backwards to her butt again. When I reached her painful area, she asked me to stay still. As I did that, I could not help noticing her moaning and groaning. At first I thought that I was hurting her, but she was quick to explain that it wasn't the case. In fact, the opposite was true. The pressure of my tiny feet on her aching back made her pain subside. After it was all over, she paid me and asked if I could come again the next day.

Later I realized that the reason she picked me was not for my good looks but for being a lightweight person. I was a skinny boy and didn't weigh very much. The lady kept asking for me and I was happy to do it. It was an easy job and I was getting paid for it. Every day after school I would go to her home and walk on top of her back. Apparently, it worked very well. To my great amazement one day, her pain was gone. I was astonished. All I did was walk on her back, doing a balancing act to keep myself from falling on top of her. I felt very proud of myself for being part of her healing process.

Imagine you are a teenager and you already discovered a way to make pain go away. I was pleased with my discovery and wanted very much to know as much as possible about it. The sad truth was that there was nobody I knew that had any knowledge about the subject of massage. I didn't understand at the time, but it seemed like when I stood on certain points for a little while, the pain subsided tremendously. Today we call those spots pressure points, but at that time, who knew? She used to say things like, "Walk slowly, a little bit to the left, now a little bit to the right. Yes, yes, that's the spot. Now stay there and don't move till I tell you," and so on.

I realize now that the experience with this sweet neighbor of mine was in fact my first introduction to massage. That experience peaked my curiosity. It gave me a great sense of satisfaction to think that my pressure on someone's back could ease her pain and make her feel so good. It was very rewarding by itself. I started asking my mother and other people I knew if they would let me practice on them. The feedback I got was encouraging, and that's how my passion for massage started.

A few years later, I enrolled in my first massage course. Unfortunately, unlike today it was not a hands-on course. Can you imagine learning massage without practising it? Right now it does not sound right. It was a different time, though. No one had heard about massage schools, like we have today. Nevertheless, I got to know some of the massage strokes from that course and how to apply them.

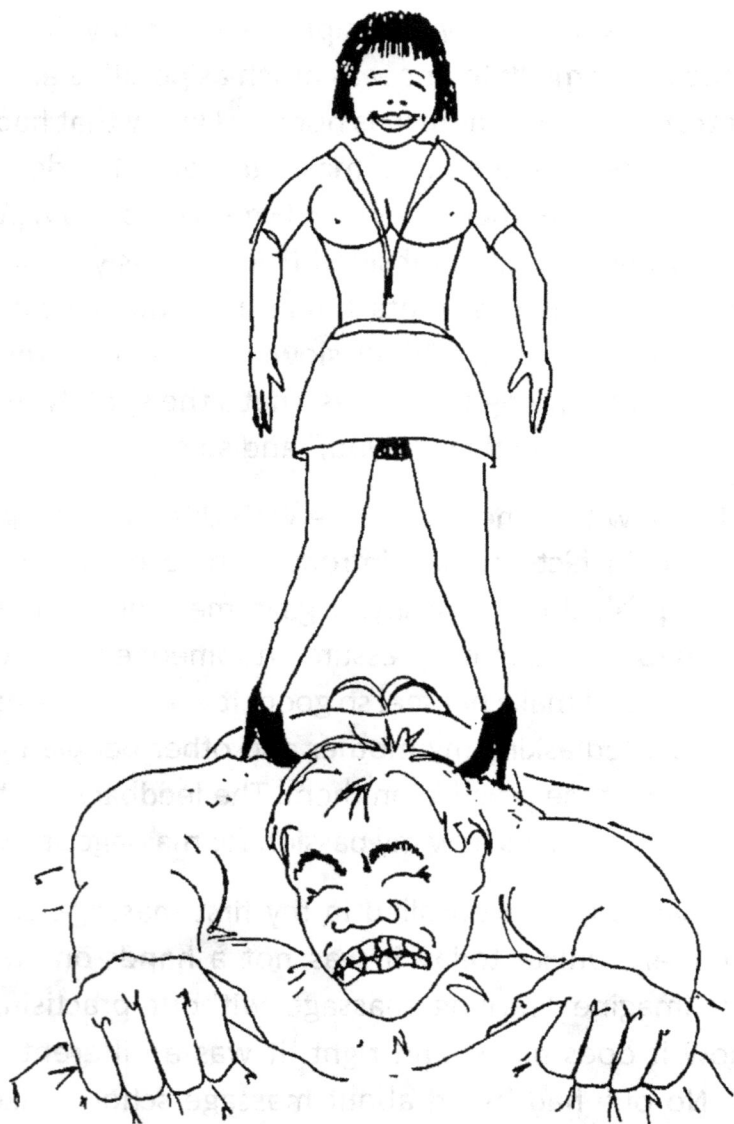

I-1

THE PRACTICE OF WALKING ON SOMEONE'S BACK IS STILL BEING USED TODAY IN ASIA.

A few years afterward, I was drafted into the military service, where I served as a medic. Whenever possible, I employed local massage, primarily for sports-related injuries of the back and neck. Subsequently, in the United States I enrolled in a well-known massage school. That was a serious course. Not only that we practised massage hands-on on each other, but we also took lots of classes in anatomy and physiology, as well as tests and licensing. I had a great love for this craft and I was determined to listen and absorb every little thing that was said and done. My mission was to be the best I could be doing it. I can tell you now that it was time well spent. Before I even graduated from massage school, I started working with a local chiropractor. That chiropractor came one day to my school and asked for a good massage therapist, and I was recommended. During the years I worked with him, he shared his knowledge and his wisdom with me, and I was grateful. From him I expanded my knowledge and took numerous seminars and courses, especially in neuromuscular massage and deep probing, specializing in pain relief methods.

I found out that during the time you spend massaging somebody, he or she may tell you a lot about their life. As a result, I became a better listener. I feel that close listening is a major skill that many of us need to develop, no matter what profession we are in. Besides, it contributes to the overall relaxation of the one receiving the massage. When you allow him or her to "unload," you have a more relaxed person on the table. I was delighted to hear from my patients over and over that out of all the treatments they were receiving in the chiropractor's office, massage helped them the most. Many of them said the only reason they were coming to the office was because they knew they were going to receive a massage as a part of their treatment.

I hope that you too, will enjoy this book and that you will put it to good use.

CHAPTER - 1
Introduction

How often have you heard, "My aching back is killing me, would you mind massaging it for me?" I'm sure you would have loved to help, if you only knew how. You just were not sure how to start? Where to start? What kind of strokes to use? How much pressure to exert? What kind of rhythm to use? Should you be fast or slow, etc.?

With the help of this book though, you will soon be able to give a satisfying massage that will help remove tension and stress and leave your partner totally relaxed. You are going to experience the sheer pleasure of making someone feel good and pain free.

Massage is an ancient practice. It has been an effective stress buster and pain reliever for thousands of years.

In addition to the obvious physical benefits, massage has psychological benefits as well. The human touch is known to reduce depression and anxiety.

From the moment we enter the world, we crave to be touched and to be stroked. It is one of the most basic and strongest human needs. Mothers instinctively and naturally massage their babies without even thinking about it. They pet, stroke, hug, and rub their babies for comfort and reassurance. In other words, massage has a nurturing effect.

Those cravings for being touched and stroked never disappear throughout our lives. It does not diminish with age and it may even intensify. It is a condition that is entirely natural. We are social creatures and have been created that way. Our bodies continue to crave both physical and emotional strokes.

The Benefits of Massage

Some of the many health benefits of receiving a massage are:

1. Relieves pain of bodily injuries.

2. Increases range of motion. After receiving a massage, we become more limber, more flexible, and maneuver better.

3. Stimulates blood circulation. Massage has a tendency to open blockages and remove impurities from our bodies. As a result, the blood moves through the veins better and gives us this tremendous high feeling that we can't help noticing after a good massage.

4. Relieves arthritic pain.

5. Prevents bed sores for those who are bedridden for a long duration of time, such as after a surgery or long illness.

6. Accelerates the healing of broken bones after the removal of a cast.

7. Aids in the treatment of internal ailments such as constipation, indigestion, bronchitis, and asthma.

8. Can help insomnia sufferers sleep better.

9. Can bring relief to those suffering from TMJ pain, (temporal mandible joints; pain in the jaws). This massage is done with a glove in the inside the mouth.

10. Can help with headaches and whiplash pain.

11. Reduces swelling of edema.

12. Delivers more oxygen to the cells.

13. Helps break the mucosa in congested patients, using cupping strokes.

14. Stimulates the flow of the lymphatic system.

15. Reduces spasms and cramping.

16. Massage can be used for pleasure and just to feel good.

Massage can be given with one of two goals in mind: either to stimulate or to relax and subdue.

To Stimulate. If, for example, you are participating in a sporting event, such as swimming, running, or boxing and you want your muscles to fire up and deliver maximum performance, this can be achieved by receiving a sports massage. Sports massage consists of rapid striking on the legs, buttocks, and upper back.

To Relax and Relieve Pain. This is what most people use massage for. The most commonly used method to achieve this goal is known as Swedish massage. This method was developed by a Swedish fencing instructor named Per Hendrik Ling in the 1830s. Mr. Ling injured his elbow one day, and he managed to heal himself by a series of strokes that he used on himself. He later expanded on it and developed this technique that is known as Swedish massage. It is also the most commonly used massage method in the United States. Unlike drug therapy that has long term side effects, massage therapy is relatively safe. It has very little contraindications and many benefits instead. The strokes in this therapy are all directed toward the heart. The main objectives are to achieve a great sense of relaxation, to relieve pain, to soothe, and to deliver more oxygen to the cells.

Some people like to believe that massage can help them lose cellulite and weight. Unfortunately, it's a myth. Massage may help break up the fat, but you still have to work on losing the weight through eating less and exercise.

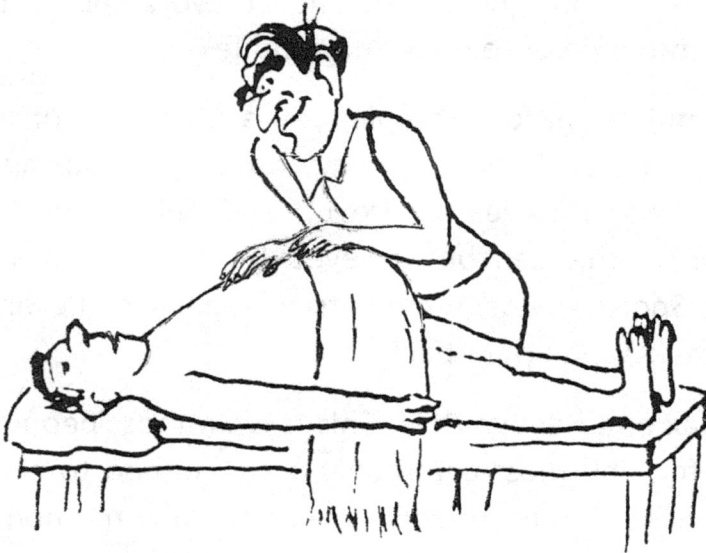

I-2

"WILL YOU PLEASE MASSAGE MY LITTLE BELLY AWAY?"

Quite a few people get up in the middle of the night and raid their refrigerator, eating whatever is inside. Since they mostly are half asleep, they either don't remember doing it or they're in denial about doing it. Sometime later when reality sets in, they call to ask if a massage will make all that extra fat disappear. If I could only say "yes" and actually deliver on this promise, I would be a very wealthy man.

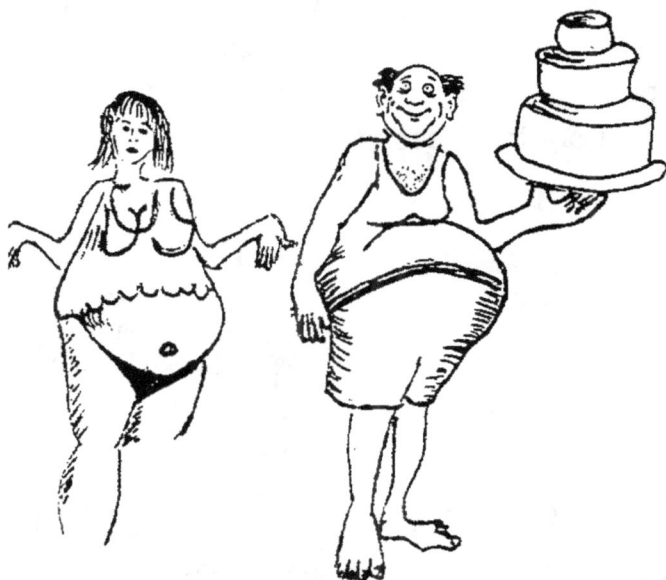

I-3

"HOW ABOUT A MIDNIGHT SNACK, HONEY?"

The Different Types of Massage

This book focuses mainly on Swedish massage, but not exclusively. Nevertheless, you should know there are other types of massage out there. Some of the best known are:

Neuromuscular Re- education. This pain relief method is achieved by pressing on the origin and insertion of muscles. This kind of massage penetrates deeper and may be more invasive than Swedish massage, but it's recommended for those who suffer from serious pain and tightness in the muscles.

Reflexology. This is a foot massage. It gives a great sense of relaxation, while at the same time stimulating healing of the body organs. Imagine that your feet are a map of your body, with lots of pressure points all over them. The pressure on those points on the bottom of the feet can speed healing to the corresponding areas of the body.

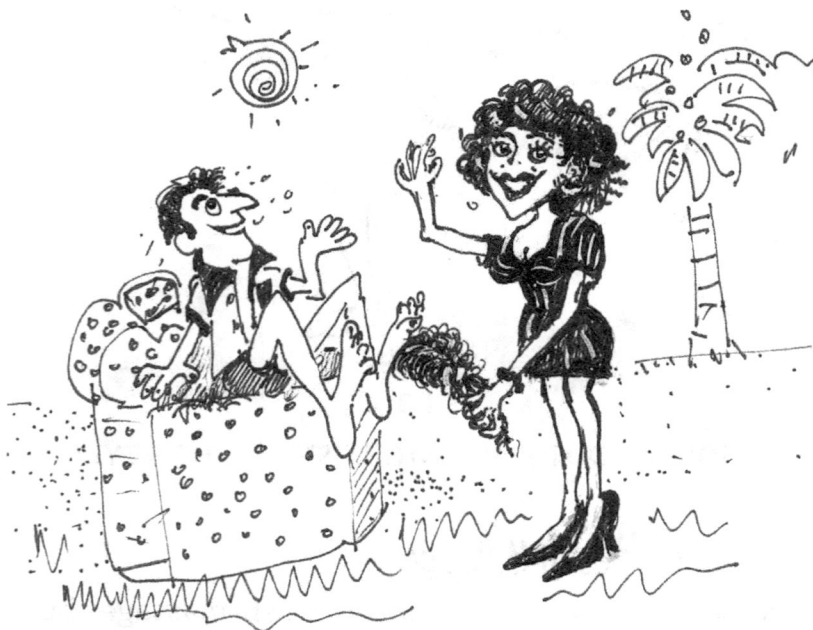

I-4

REFLEXOLOGY IS A FOOT MASSAGE.
YOU APPLY PRESSURE MAINLY WITH YOUR THUMBS TO CERTAIN POINTS ON THE FEET.

Rolfing. This is probably the most painful massage technique that I know of. Rolfing was developed by Doctor Ida Rolf in the 1920's. The goal of Rolfing is structural integration alignment. It means to align the human structure in balance with gravity. Structural integration can be effective in relieving chronic pain such as back pain, scoliosis, sciatica, tense muscles, and carpel tunnel syndrome. For some, this kind of bodywork may trigger an emotional release (such as sobbing and crying) during treatment.

Shiatsu. The Japanese are famous for this style of massage. The word *shiatsu* means "finger pressure." The goal of shiatsu is to achieve a balanced energy flow within the body.

Sports Massage. This type of massage is usually given to athletes who compete in sports. Sports massage has two parts to it. The first part is given just before the sporting event to stimulate the muscles to deliver maximum performance. The stroke mainly used to do so is called tapotement (rapid striking). The second part is given after the sporting event is over, when the body needs to come down from a hyper state to a normal relaxed state.

Although we will not be discussing these other techniques in detail, it is important to know of their existence. This book is written mainly for those who wish to practise massage to give soothing, relaxing massage for the purpose of pleasure, relaxation, and some pain relief. Knowing how to give a good massage will give a person an edge socially. It is certainly a topic of conversation and invites feelings of warmth and closeness. Massage brings about and enhances intimacy with one's mate, and it is important to note that the giver should be a receiver as well. This is the best way for the giver to feel firsthand how the strokes actually feel. I encourage both partners in a relationship to learn the techniques in this book, because everyone deserves a good massage.

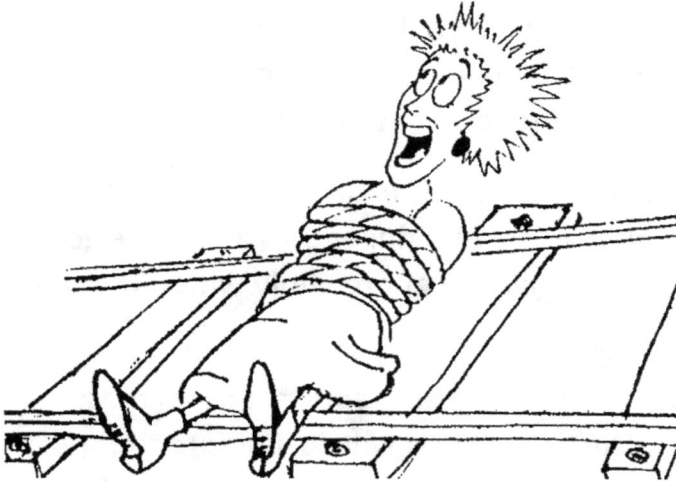

I-5

"AHH…THE STRESS OF EVERYDAY LIFE…CAN MAKE YOU SCREAM FOR A GOOD MASSAGE."

Who Can Have a Massage?

You can massage anyone with reasonably good health. Massage should not be given to someone with high fever, cancer, AIDS, tuberculosis, infectious diseases, open sores, varicose veins, diabetes, or blood clots.

We already know that massage makes the blood flow better in the body. When massaging someone with one of the diseases mention above, you could be helping to spread that disease even further through the blood. As the blood circulates better, so will the diseases. The golden rule is, when in doubt, get a doctor's approval. Don't take unnecessary risks. Give massage to only healthy individuals.

Tools of the Trade

You don't need much to perform a successful massage. The main tools are your hands and how you use them. Having said that, some items will make massage an easy and more pleasurable experience.

- Massage table. If you are going to give massages regularly and perhaps to more people than just your partner, a massage table can be a worthy investment. Massage tables come in many varieties; sometimes you can even purchase a secondhand table inexpensively if you look in the local newspaper. Personally, I like the lightweight tables, the kind that you can fold and put aside when the massage is over. The main benefit is that a massage table can be adjusted to your height, and this is important, as you need to protect your own back from injury. The second advantage is that it's comfortable for the person receiving the massage as it has a cutout for the face when lying on your stomach. If such a table is not available, use a strong kitchen table. If you don't have a strong table, set up for massage on the floor.

The rest of the things that you may use are:

- One bed sheet.

- Two medium - sized towels.

- One big towel.

- Massage oil or massage cream. You may find these items at a local health food store. Note: When using massage oil, make sure it's made of vegetable pressed oil.

How to Prepare a Massage Table

1. Make sure the height of the massage table is about ten inches below your belt line, so you will not pull your back out while giving the massage.

2. Spread the bed sheet on top of the massage table.

3. Spread the two medium-sized towels to form a *T* shape.

4. Place the folded beach towel on the table. Later on your subject will be using this towel to cover himself or herself prior to receiving the massage.

5. Have your massage oil close by.

6. Soft music and a nice scent are a plus, but not essential.

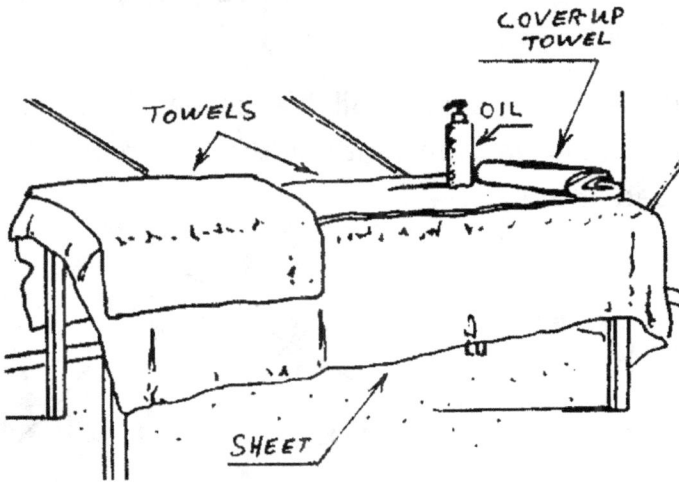

I-6

A MASSAGE TABLE SETUP

Massage on the Kitchen Table or the Floor

If you have no massage table, but your kitchen table is strong enough, set up for massage on top of the kitchen table.

Performing massage on the floor is not easy. If you have a weak back, giving a massage while you are on your hands and knees may hurt you.

Whether you are giving a massage on the kitchen table or the floor, padding is important.

1. Spread out a comforter or cushion.

2. Spread a bed sheet on top of the cushion.

3. Cross the two medium-sized towels across each other in the shape of a T.

4. Have a big beach towel handy so your partner can cover up.

If a kitchen table is not available, spread a comforter or a cushion on the floor, then continue with the rest of the setup as described above.

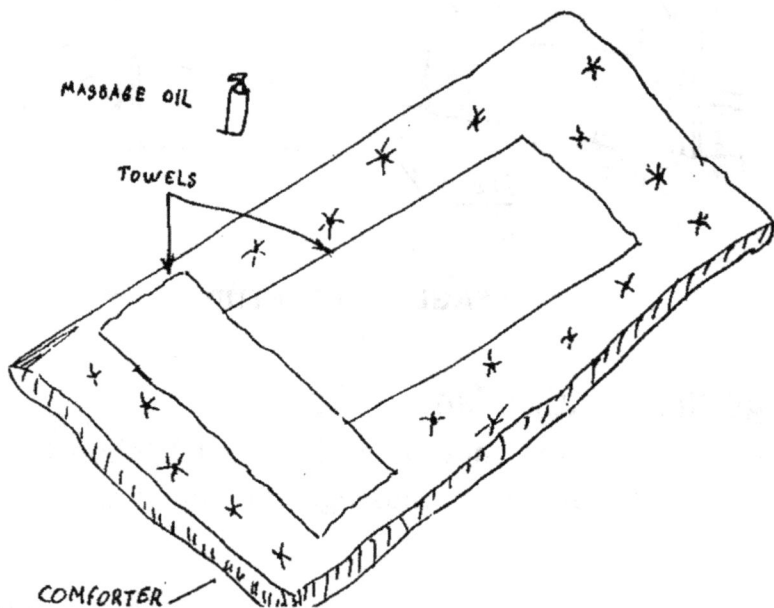

MASSAGE OIL

TOWELS

COMFORTER

I-7

MASSAGE SETUP ON THE FLOOR OR THE KITCHEN TABLE.

The Room Setting

A peaceful and safe environment is vital when it comes to keeping your partner relaxed to achieve a successful massage.

Here are some tips for selecting a good location for massage:

• The location you choose should be quiet and private. Have at least two feet of clearance around the working area. This will allow you the freedom to move around the table with ease as you work.

- Dim the lights. Harsh light may disturb the eyes and prevent your partner from enjoying the massage. Indirect lighting is best. You can add a candle for a romantic mood.

- Play soft music. It should be mellow and tranquil. If possible, select instrumental pieces, something soothing that will help your partner relax.

- Have a pleasant aroma in the room, if possible. You may choose a scented candle, incense sticks, or scented massage oil.

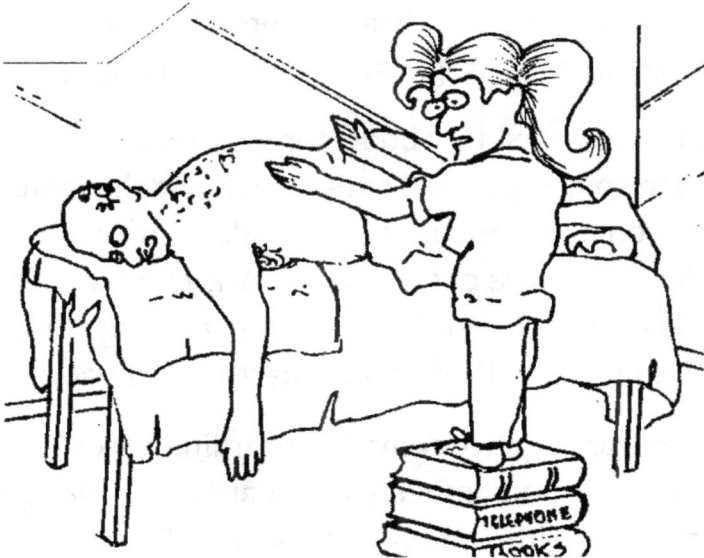

I-8

"THIS TABLE IS JUST TOO HIGH FOR ME; I NEED TO 'RISE UP' FOR THE OCCASION."

Cleanliness

It goes without saying that you should be clean when getting so close to somebody. Pay close attention to your nails. Even if they are short, they can be sharp and can cause injury to your partner during the massage. Make sure they are smooth and well rounded. If you have a cut on your finger that may bleed, you should delay giving a massage until such time as your cut has healed.

Ethics

A person may feel vulnerable without his clothes on. Respect the fact that he or she has invested in you. Don't embarrass your partner in any way; your partner will respect you for that. Uncover only the part of the body that you're working on. The rest can stay covered. A person needs to uncover less on a massage table than on the beach.

During massage, the body temperature of the person receiving the massage tends to decrease, and the temperature of the person giving the massage tends to increase, because of the physical nature of the activity. Ask your partner if he or she needs an extra cover. Don't allow strangers into the room during the massage. Protect your partner's privacy.

Don't make negative remarks regarding his or her weight or appearance. Remember your goal is to have a relaxed person to work with, not an agitated one. People come in all sizes and shapes, and none of us is perfect.

These suggestions may be common sense, but they become vitally important when a person is lying down with only a towel covering his or her naked body. Remember your partner is trusting you.

Focus on your partner and give him or her you undivided attention and sensitivity for the duration of the massage. Be alert to bruises, rashes, hard lumps, or anything that may seem medically unusual. If you spot something suspicious, bring it to your partner's attention: you can suggest that this lump or a rash better be checked by a doctor. You will be surprised how little people know about their own bodies.

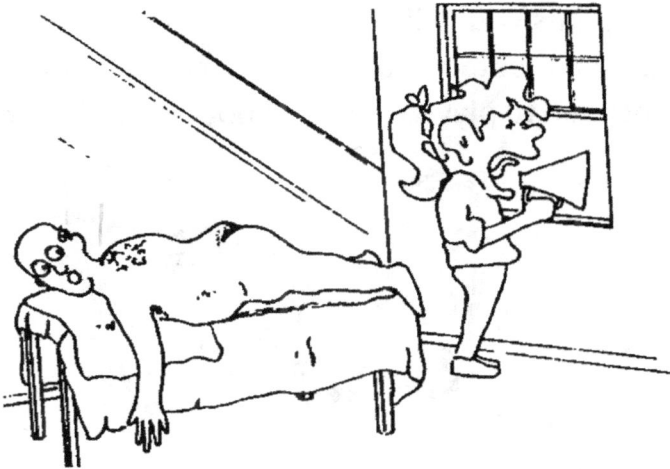

I-9

"HURRY UP AND COME OVER HERE. YOU WILL NEVER BELIEVE WHO I HAVE NAKED ON MY TABLE."

Communication

Encourage your partner to keep lines of communication open, and continue to adjust to his or her needs.

Your first question should be, "Is there any reason why you shouldn't be receiving a massage?" If the answer is no, ask, "Is there any special area you want me to concentrate on?"

Ask your partner if the pressure you are applying is too strong or too light. Pay attention to body language, such as facial and other body signals of uneasiness with your pressure. Some people may be too embarrassed to let you know you are hurting them. Body language, however, always tells the truth. Lighten up on the pressure you are applying if you see signs of discomfort. Don't assume a man can take more pressure than a woman; in fact, the opposite may be true. Many times you will discover that even a small woman can tolerate pain better than a big, muscular man. Men may be more inclined to play macho and not complain about pain.

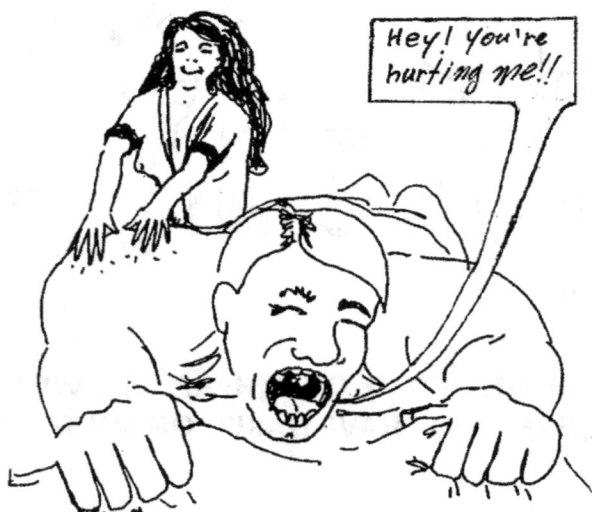

I-10

DON'T ASSUME THAT BIG MEN TOLERATE PAIN BETTER THAN A WOMAN.

CHAPTER - 2
Massage—Facing Up

You start by massaging the front of your subject first, afterwards you turn your subject over facing down and you massage the back area.

It is important not to lose focus of what you are trying to accomplish. You must do your best to help your partner relax. To do so, you must be relaxed and confident yourself. When your partner sees you relaxed and confident, he or she will feel that they are in the right hands and most likely will close their eyes and let you do your work in peace. To get into that relaxed state of mind, take a deep breathe, then hold it for a few seconds, then exhale. Try breathing through your nose and exhaling through your mouth. Repeat this exercise three times. You can apply this technique not only when giving a massage but also whenever you feel nervous, such as when you are sitting in a dentist's chair waiting for someone to drill in your mouth, when you are waiting for an important interview, and so on.

Count on forty-five minutes to an hour for a full body massage.

Massage Strokes

You should be familiar with several types of massage strokes in order to perform an effective massage. It will take a little time to master them, but with a little practice it can be done. We will get into the details of each stroke as we progress, and you will learn how to use each and every stroke, as well as the sequence.

When giving Swedish massage, all strokes move toward the heart. The strokes are also much more effective when performed slowly and in a soothing manner. You can't rush through the act of administering massage.

Effleurage. This is the most commonly used stroke. If you forget everything else, remember how to do effleurage, it is simply a gliding stroke with open palms. We use it to smooth the muscles and to relax the nerves; we also use this stroke to apply oil. While doing this stroke, you may be able to feel spasms and knots under the skin surface. That's why effleurage is also known as the evaluation stroke. Effleurage is also an in-between stroke. We use it whenever we change from one kind of stroke to another.

To perform it properly, simply place your palms flat on the skin surface, apply pressure, and let your palms glide from one end of the body part you are massaging to the other end of it. Never do an incomplete stroke. Your partner may feel that he is getting cheated and not getting what has been promised.

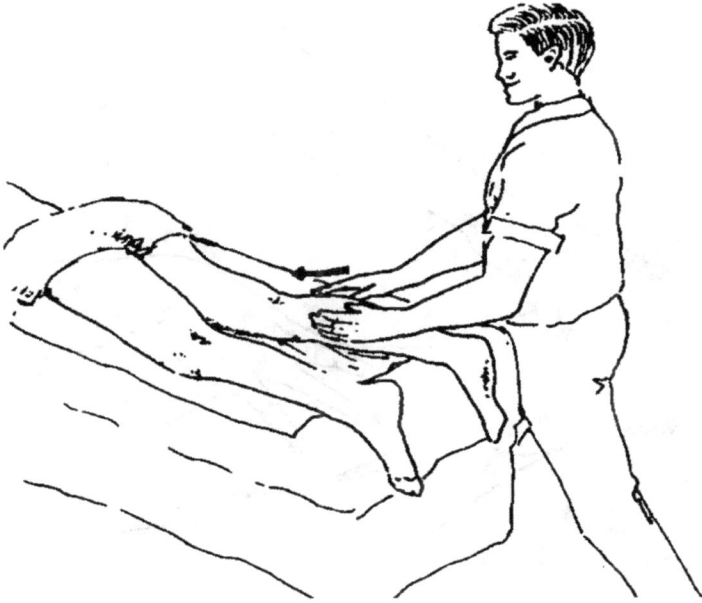

I-11

**EFFLEURAGE—PRESS YOUR PALMS
AGAINST THE SKIN TISSUE AND GLIDE.**

If you feel you need to reach the deeper layer of the muscle tissue, you may perform effleurage with your fingertips. Simply place your fingertips against the muscle tissue, apply pressure, and glide.

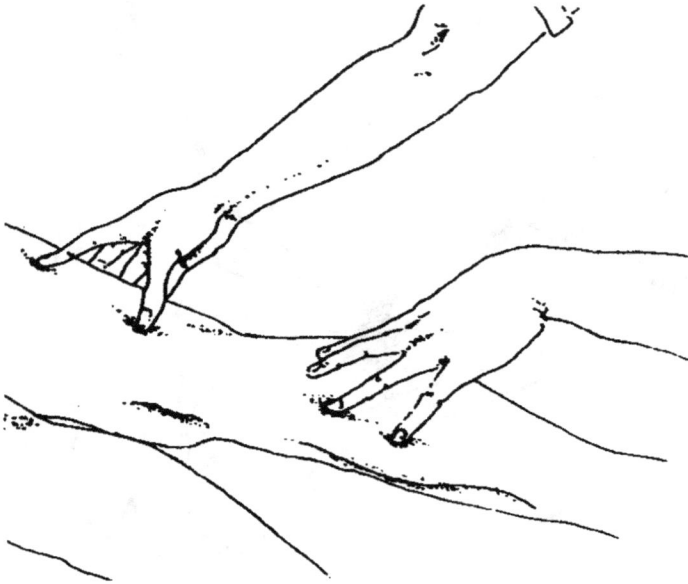

I-12

**FOR DEEP EFFLEURAGE, USE STIFF FINGERS
FOR A DEEPER PENETRATION.**

Petrissage. This is similar to kneading or "milking" the muscle tissue. Make a *C* formation with each palm and place your hands on the body part you want to massage. Pass the muscle tissue mass from one hand to the other, without pinching.

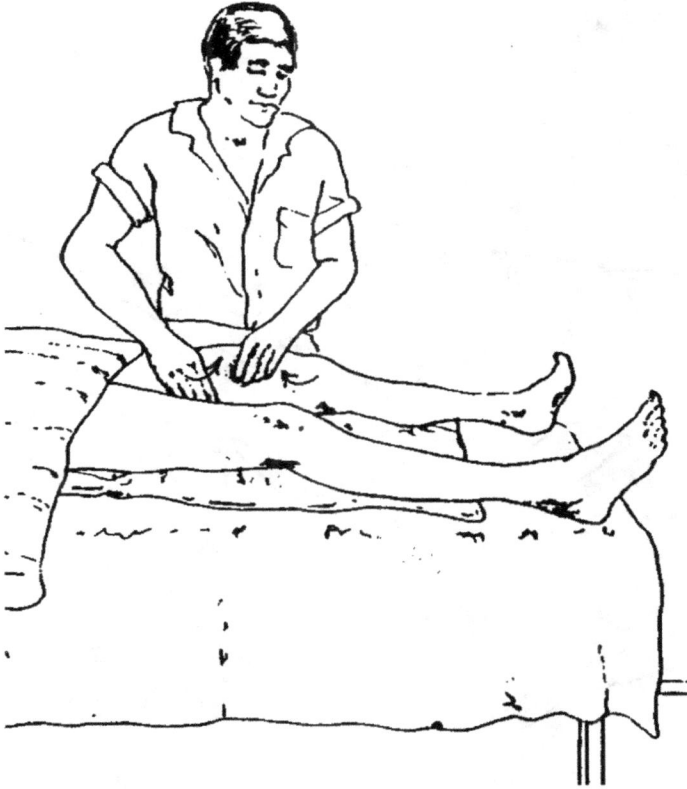

I-13

PETRISSAGE—SQUEEZE GENTLY, LIFT, AND PASS THE MUSCLE FROM ONE HAND TO ANOTHER.

Friction. Friction is compressing and moving the underlying tissue. Friction is an effective action to loosen adhesions and to separate the muscle's fiber.

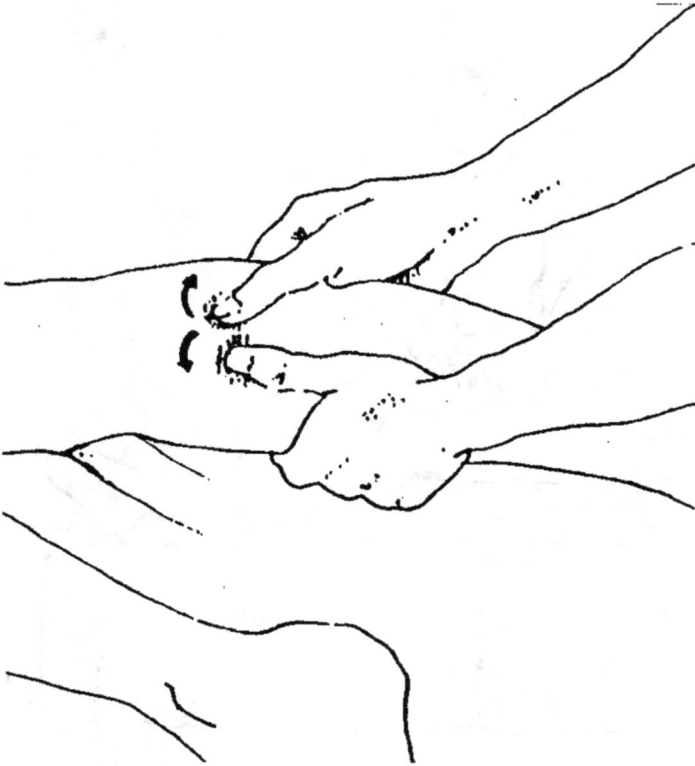

I-14

**FRICTION—IT'S A DEEP THUMB PRESSURE
WITH RIGHT AND LEFT MOTIONS.**

Vibration. Vibration is an oscillatory movement given to loosen a certain body part. For this technique, place your stiff fingers onto the muscle tissue and quickly vibrate and shake the muscle tissue left and right, left and right.

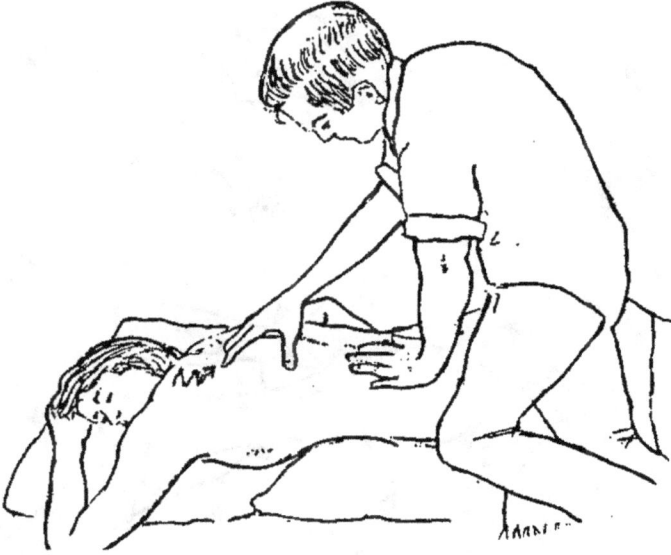

1-15

VIBRATION-PRESS YOUR FINGERS ONTO THE MUSCLE TISSUE AND MAKE A SHAKING MOTION.

Tapotement. It is a rapid striking of the muscle. Tapotement is generally used in sport massage for stimulation purposes and is done using open hands and loose fingers, like hitting a drum with a karate chops. Perform this stroke by striking with the pinky edge of your hand very quickly. It is an excellent stroke to use before running, swimming, biking, or other sporting events.

Never use tapotement over the kidney (lower back) or the stomach.

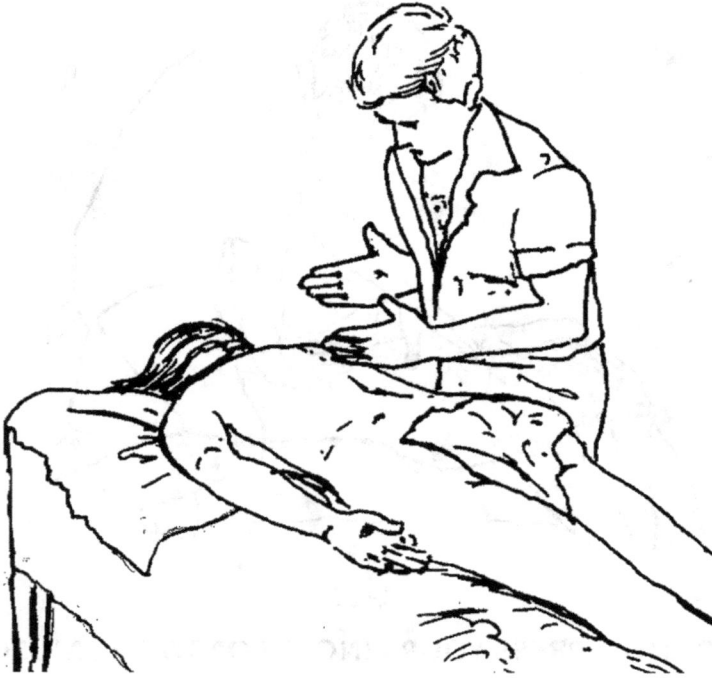

I-16

TAPOTEMENT—A RAPID STRIKING.

Speaking from my experience, most people don't like to receive tapotement. It feels like someone is beating up on them (but it certainly looks good in the movies, doesn't it?).

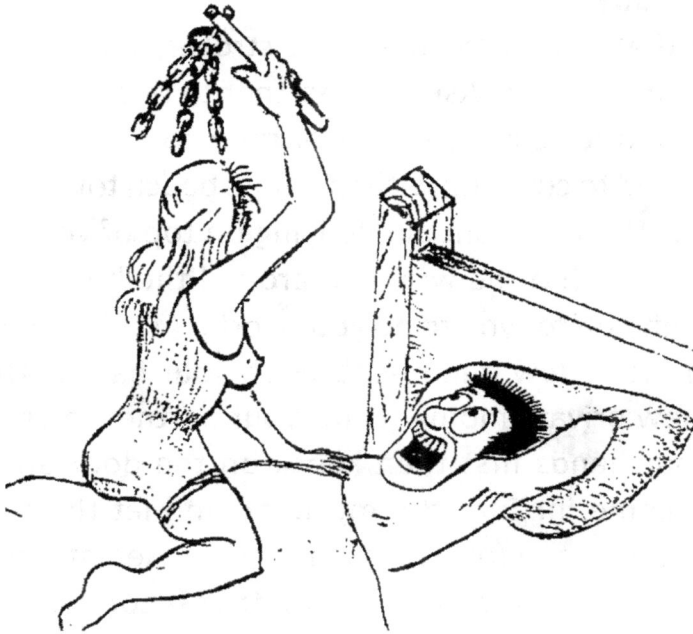

I-17

"WOW! YOU TAKE YOUR TAPOTEMENT VERY SERIOUSLY."

Nerve Strokes. Every once in awhile, I like to adopt a new stroke and add it to my massage routine. In this case it is nerve stroke. This one is not part of the Swedish massage per se. Nerve strokes show completion of work on a particular body part. These strokes consist of light touches. It is done with your fingertips by barely touching the skin and the hair follicles of the body part you are stroking. This stroke is pleasant, soothing, and pampering.

When performing all the strokes mentioned above, try to achieve continuity, or a flow to your motions. It takes a little practice, but it will become easier with each massage you perform.

Getting Ready

Now that you know the basic strokes, it's time to get ready to apply them. Ask your partner to remove his or her clothing and jewelry. Ask your partner to lie down (facing upward) and to cover up with the large beach towel that you provided. The towel should be lying on top of your subject like a blanket, (not be wrapped around the body, as it will make it difficult for you to do your work). At this point, leave the room for a few minutes to wash your hands. That will leave a few private moments for your partner to get ready. Wash your hands first then knock on the door and ask if you can come in. Turn the music on and let the soothing sound set the tone for a pleasant and relaxed atmosphere. Dim the light, making sure your partner is comfortable and relaxed.

Remember, once you establish physical contact; try not to break it until you are all done with your massage. As we discussed earlier, massage has a nurturing effect. Your partner will come to rely on your touch for the duration of the massage. Most people like to have their eyes closed when they are receiving a massage. Sometimes they will be facing down, so you know that as far as they are concerned you are there as they feel your touch. Lifting your hands off their body could be interpreted as a sign of neglect or that you have left the room.

It is not that hard to maintain contact with your partner for the duration of the massage. For example, if you are applying massage oil or cream to your hands, make a cup shape with your hand and let it rest on the body part you are massaging. That will leave your other hand free to add the oil onto the hand resting on the body part that you are massaging. Rub your hands together while maintaining a casual contact and continue massaging your subject.

Here is another example of how not to break a contact during massage. Suppose you want to move from one side of your table to the other side. Just briefly touch your partner on your way to the new location. This will reassure him or her that you did not leave the room and you are still engaged.

Massage Sequence

Facing Up. When your partner is facing up, begin the massage with the head, moving to the neck and shoulders, then hands and fingers, and ending with the legs and feet.

Facing Down. When your partner is facing down, begin with the legs and feet, moving to the neck and shoulders, and ending with the back.

Where to Start

As shown in our massage sequence above, start by massaging the head, then the neck and shoulders. These areas accumulate lots of stress and tension. Once you relax these areas, the rest of the body will most likely surrender itself to you. Remind your partner to remain as loose and relaxed as possible to experience the full benefits.

Some massage therapists, especially Europeans, prefer to start the massage at the feet. I prefer to do it the American way. I start with the head and gradually go down to the feet. It's also more sanitary.

Know How Much Pressure to Apply

Knowing how much pressure to apply is the hardest thing to teach. Every person that you massage will have a different preference. You can also say that each massage therapist has his or her own touch, even if they all were taught by the same teacher. It's like a signature. Each one is unique and different from anybody else.

The key is to ask, "How am I doing? Do you like deeper or lighter pressure?" In general, start light, and as you loosen the area you are working on, you can apply deeper pressure. Remember that pain responds to pressure very well.

When receiving a massage yourself, pay attention to the strokes and the pressure that are being applied to you and how they make you feel. Pay attention to each body part, as the pressure should be different in different places of the body. For example, you don't apply the same pressure massaging your partner's head as you would when massaging your partner's back. Try adopting the strokes and pressure that made you feel good to be used later upon somebody else.

Head Massage

The head is the only area to which we do not apply massage oil. The reason we use oil or cream is the same reason it is used in cars; to reduce friction. Oil makes the gliding stroke smoother and reduces friction. The head, however, is too small and too delicate for oil. The last thing you want to do is get oil or cream into your partner's eyes or into other facial cavities.

- Have your partner lie down on the table facing up.

- Stand behind your subject's head, rubbing your hands together until they are warm enough. Place them flat on your partner's face, covering most of his or her face with your palms, except for the nose. Let your partner enjoy the heat that flows from your hands into his or her face for about ten seconds.

- Apply light pressure on the forehead, and glide down with your hands from the center of the forehead toward the ears using the effleurage stroke. Repeat this movement three times.

- Now place your thumbs on each side of the nose tip and glide them gently toward the eye sockets.

- When you reach the points where the nose meets the eye sockets, hold pressure on these points with your thumbs for thirty seconds. Repeat that twice. These pressure points help open the drainage of the nasal cavity and reduce headaches caused by congestion.

Refer to the following illustration for the location of these pressure points.

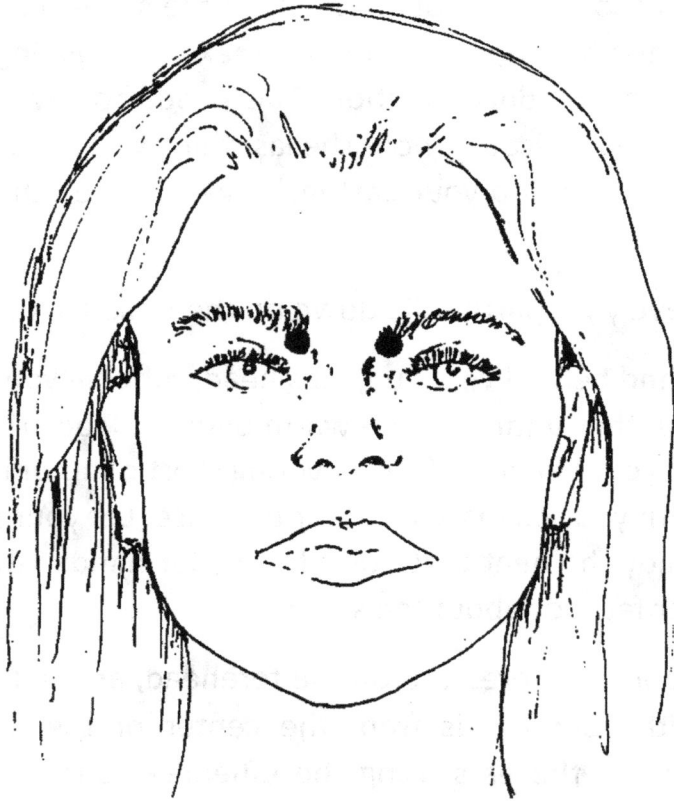

I-18

PRESSURE POINTS FOR HEADACHE RELIEF CAUSED BY STUFFINESS IN THE SINUS CAVITIES.

- Now place your thumbs flat on the cheeks beside the nose.

- Stroke the cheeks gently toward the ears with the effleurage stroke as shown in the next illustration. Two repetitions are sufficient.

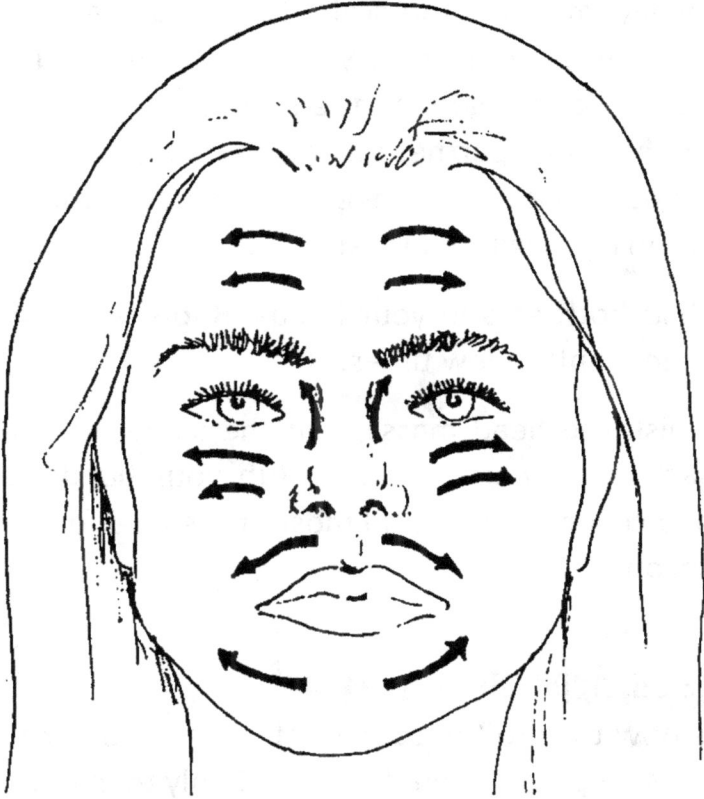

I-19

STROKE DIRECTIONS WHEN DOING FACIAL MASSAGE.

- Use the same stroke with your thumbs to do the mustache area (between the upper lip and the nose). Repeat twice.

- Now use the same stroke over the chin as well. Place your thumbs on top of the chin and glide toward the ears in two repetitions. All of these strokes are performed mainly with the thumbs using the effleurage technique.

- Finally, massage the scalp. Scalp massage is relaxing and enjoyable, so take your time with it. Put the ten tips of your fingers on the scalp and pretend you are washing your partner's hair with shampoo. Use circular motions with your fingers as well as some pressure when massaging the scalp.

- Hold both ears in your hands. Rub them and wiggle them gently a few times.

- Finish the head massage at the same place and the same way you started it. Rub your hands together and cover the eyes and most of the face for about ten seconds.

Massage Oil, Application

Let's now turn to the subject of massage oil or massage cream. First apply it to your hands and only then to the body. Place a small amount of massage oil in one palm. Rub your hands together until it's evenly distributed on both hands and apply it to the body. Apply oil only to the aria on which you are working one part at a time. Do not apply too much oil to avoid getting messy, as well as losing your grip.

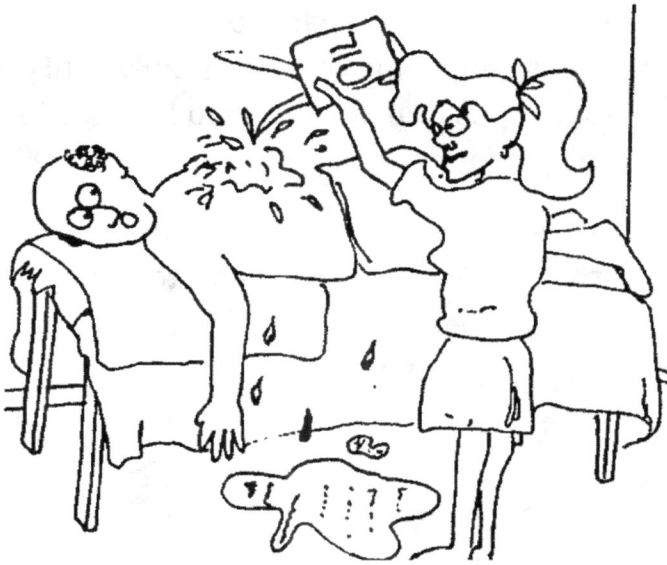

I-20

APPLY ONLY A SMALL AMOUNT OF OIL AT A TIME.

Neck and Shoulder Massage

- While standing behind your partner's head, place your open hands on each side of the upper arms. Apply pressure, and glide your hands slowly toward the shoulders and the neck.

- While you are doing this, change your hands from open palms into fists, while moving your fists toward the neck. Don't be afraid to apply pressure. This pressure feels good, especially on the upper shoulders and neck.

- Continue gliding your fists gently toward the neck until your two fists meet each other under the neck.

- On the way back, glide back to the shoulders and the upper arms, reopening your fists slowly until you return to the same position at which you started. Repeat this stroke about four times.

This stroke may be a little difficult to master at first, but performing it well will reduce pain and tension in the neck and shoulders. The next three illustrations will give you a better understanding of how to perform it.

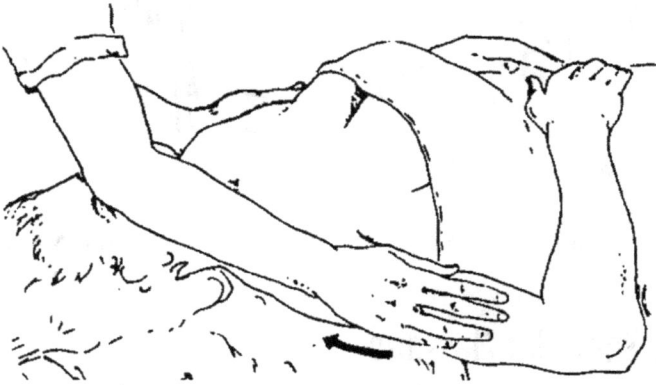

I-21

PLACE YOUR HANDS ON THE UPPER ARM, PRESS AND GLIDE TOWARD THE NECK.

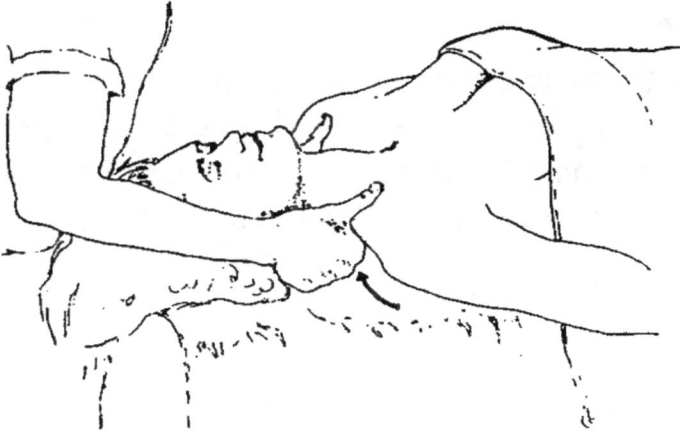

I-22

WHILE MOVING TOWARD THE NECK, TRANSFORM YOUR OPEN PALMS TO FISTS.

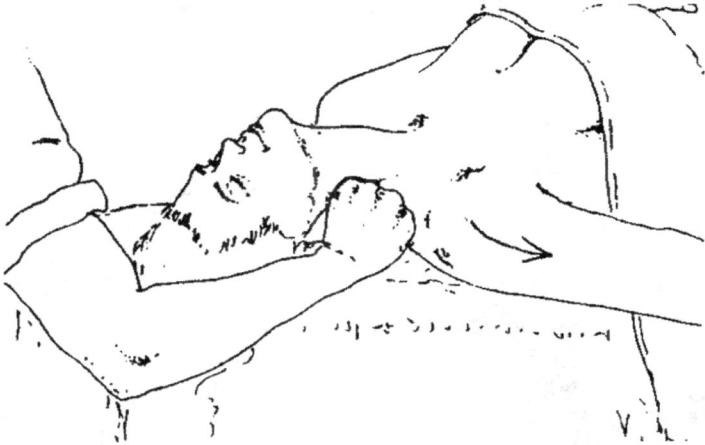

I-23

START RELEASING THE PRESSURE ON THE SHOULDERS.

OPEN YOUR FISTS AND GLIDE BACK TO THE UPPER ARM, YOUR STARTING POINT.

Neck Stretching

Neck stretching can loosen the tightness in the neck, upper back, and shoulders, as well as the arms. Note: Even though stretching is not part of massage, it can be a great contributor to the overall relaxation of the body.

- Place both hands under the head and turn the head sideways very gently.

- Place one of your hands at the base of the skull and the other on top of your partner's shoulder. Apply pressure in the opposite direction and hold that pressure for about thirty seconds.

- Now turn the head gently to the other side and do the same to that side.

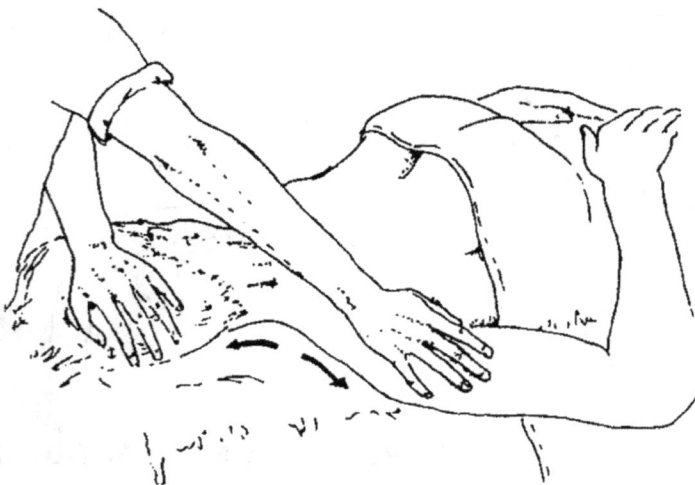

I-24

PLACE ONE HAND ON THE BASE OF THE SKULL AND THE OTHER ON THE SHOULDER,

THEN STRETCH IN THE OPPOSITE DIRECTION.

Arm and Shoulder Strokes

- Release the pressure on the neck while maintaining support of the head with one of your hands.

- Place your other hand flat on the upper arm close to the elbow.

- Now glide it toward the neck. At the same time change from a flat palm to a fist.

- Glide with your fist all the way to the base of the skull

- On the way back, release some of the pressure, open your fist slowly, and glide back till you reach the elbow—your starting point. Repeat this stroke back and forth three times.

- Once you are done with that side, support the head with two hands and move it gently to the opposite side. Now you can do the same stroke on the other side as well.

- Afterwards, move the head gently to the center position.

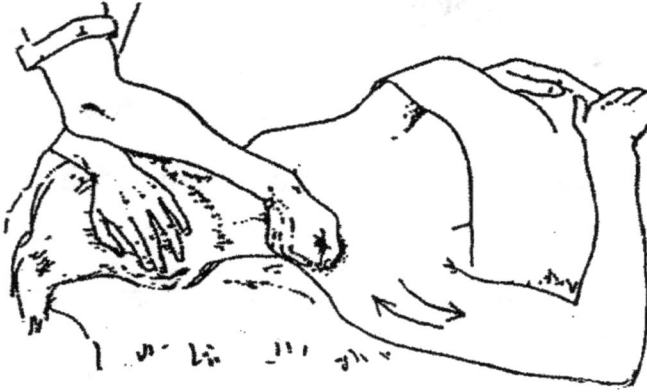

I-25

START WITH YOUR PALM FLAT ON THE UPPER ARM. GLIDE UPWARDS TOWARD THE HEAD.

WHILE DOING SO TRANSFORM YOUR PALM TO FIST. ON THE WAY BACK, OPEN YOUR FIST SLOWLY

AND GLIDE TILL YOU REACH YOUR STARTING POINT BY THE ELBOW.

Pay attention to the fact that you have just finished stretching the neck as well as massaging the arm and shoulder on one side. Both of those actions were done while the head was slightly tilted to one side. Now it's time for you to lift the head gently from that position and tilt the head to the opposite side. In order to balance the body, you should do exactly the same stretch to the other side.

Neck Massage

- Apply very little oil to your hands.

- Try forming a cup shape with your palms as shown in the next illustration.

- Place your hands on both sides of the neck and perform deep strokes with the tips of your fingers. Start where the shoulders meet the neck and stroke the neck toward the hairline. To do this right you should lift the head an inch or two from the massage table.

- Alternate with your hands, left, right, left, right, about six strokes with each hand.

Keep your nails short to avoid risking injury to your partner. If you are not careful, your nails can cut right through the back of the neck.

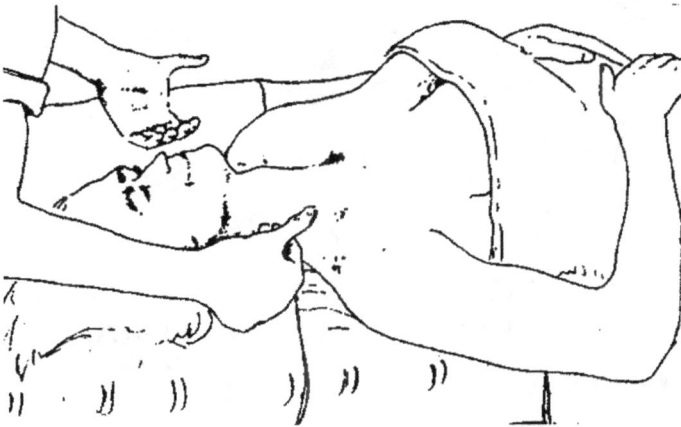

I-26

PLACE YOUR HANDS UNDER THE NECK AND STROKE IT TOWARD YOU. LEFT, RIGHT, LEFT, RIGHT...

The Body Mechanics Technique

When working on a long stretch of body, such as a leg or hand, the risk of injuring your own back increases. The solution to this problem is to practise what is known in the trade as body mechanics. This can be accomplished by moving your own body in the same direction of the stroke. By doing so your back remains straight at all times.

If you ever saw a massage therapist at work, he might appear light on his feet, like a skillful dancer.

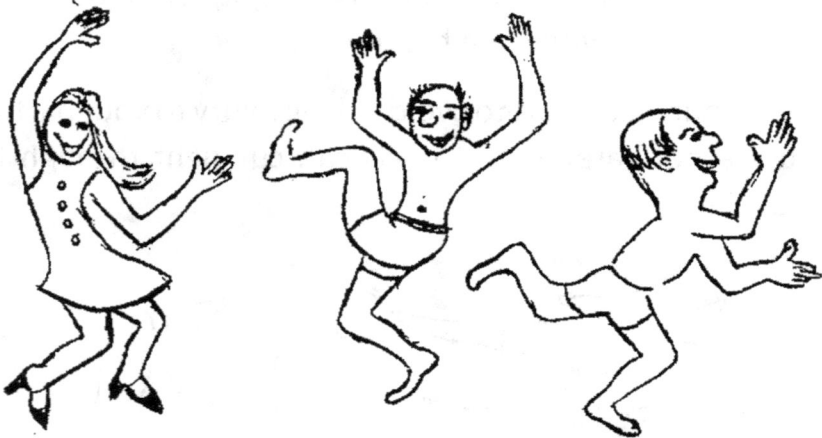

I-27

THE PRACTICE OF BODY MECHANICS TECHNIQUE CAN SAVE YOU FROM INJURY.

Massaging the Arm

- Stand by the side of your partner, next to one of his arms. Spread your legs shoulder-width apart to achieve good stability.

- Apply massage cream or oil to your palms. Rub them together, and spread the oil evenly to cover your partner's arm from the wrist to the shoulder.

- Secure the hand you are massaging by placing one of your palms on top of your partner's palm. With your other hand, press your palm close to the wrist and glide along the entire arm with an effleurage stroke. Apply more pressure on the way up to the shoulder.

- On the way down to the palm, reduce pressure on the arm. Repeat this stroke about four times while using the body mechanics technique.

Note: A general rule that can be used for all strokes is: Apply pressure when moving toward the heart and reduce pressure when moving away from the heart.

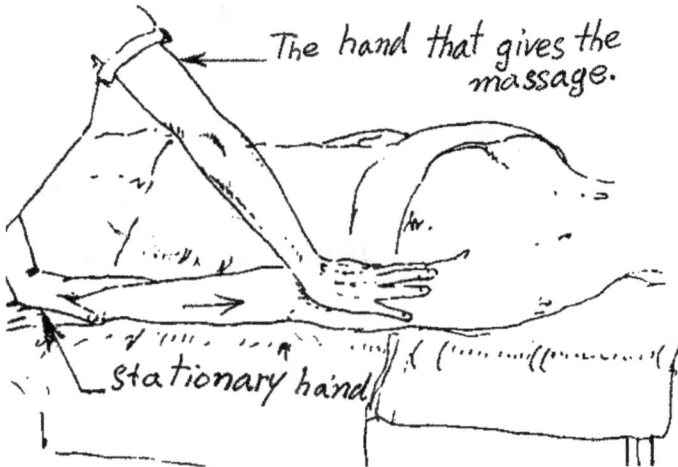

I-28

EFFLEURAGE STROKE, OVER THE ARM.

Palm Massage

- Lift your partner's palm and support it with one of your hands.

- Now make a fist with your other hand and stroke with your fist and knuckles onto the inside of your partner's palm for about five repetitions.

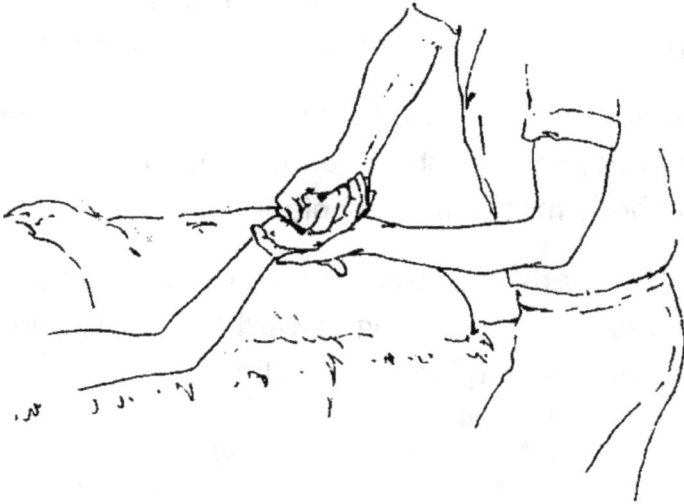

I-29

MAKE A FIST AND MASSAGE THE INSIDE OF THE PALM.

- Stretch the palm by pulling and spreading it with both of your hands.

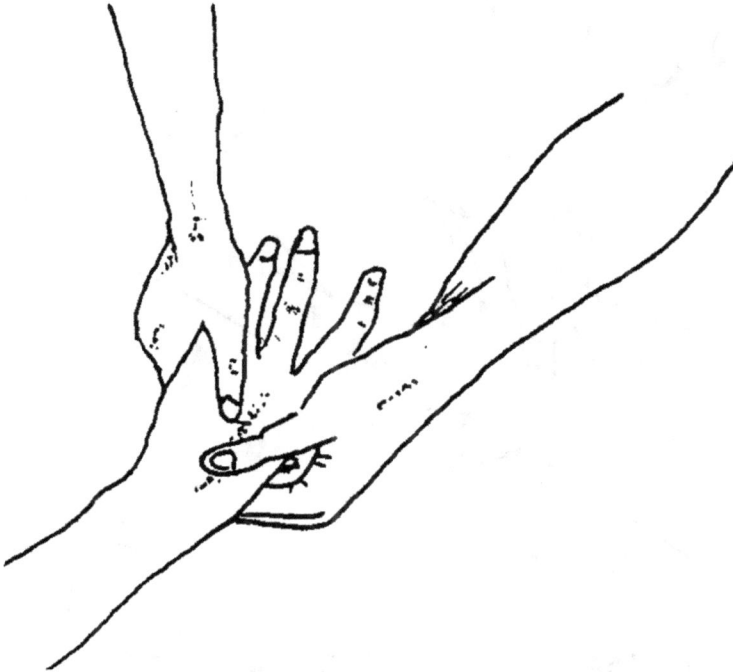

I-30

STRETCH AND SPREAD THE PALM.

- You are going to massage the area between the wrist and the fingers, on the outside portion of your partner's palm.

- Place your thumbs between the bony areas and massage the soft tissue between them. You can do this using your thumbs, one thumb following another, using the friction stroke. Remember, we don't massage bones, just the soft tissue between them.

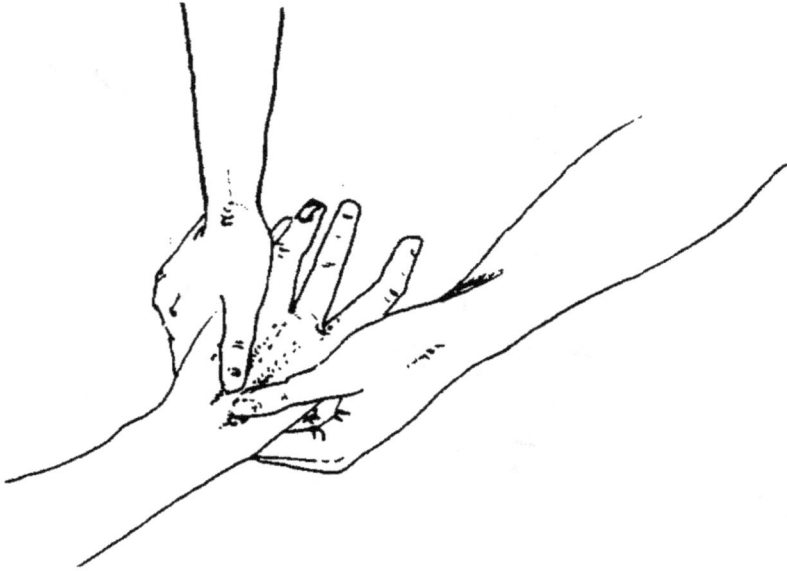

I-31

**MASSAGE WITH YOUR THUMBS BETWEEN
THE BONY AREAS OF YOUR PARTNER'S PALM.**

Fingers Massage

- Take each finger between your thumb and index finger and "milk it" (gently pulling and gliding, such as when milking a cow).

- As you approach the end of each finger, give it a little squeeze on the nail area.

- Rub the area between the fingers as well, using your thumb and index finger.

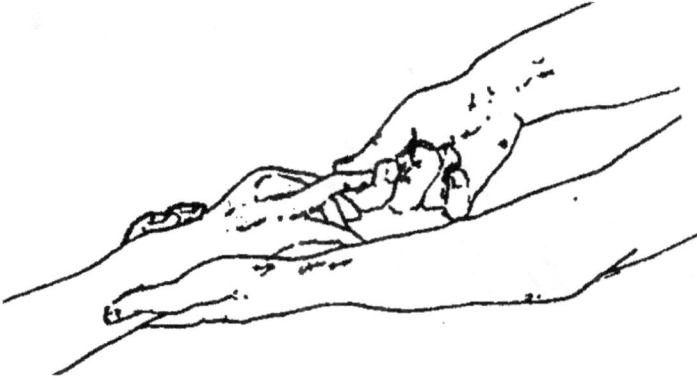

I-32

"MILK" EACH FINGER GENTLY BETWEEN YOUR THUMB AND INDEX FINGER.

- Effleurage the whole arm again, as shown in I-28. Lift the forearm gently with one of your hands and "milk" it, from the wrist to the elbow in petrissage fashion or C formation. That C shape is being formed between your thumb and index finger (see illustration I-26) as discussed earlier.

- Repeat that twice, then switch sides and do the other hand the same way.

Remember, when doing petrissage, you pass the muscle tissue from one hand to another. This one is an exception though. The stroke is still petrissage stroke, but since you are supporting the wrist with one of your hands, you have some limitations. You must do this stroke with one hand only like milking with one hand. For instance, squeeze, push forward, let go, and so forth.

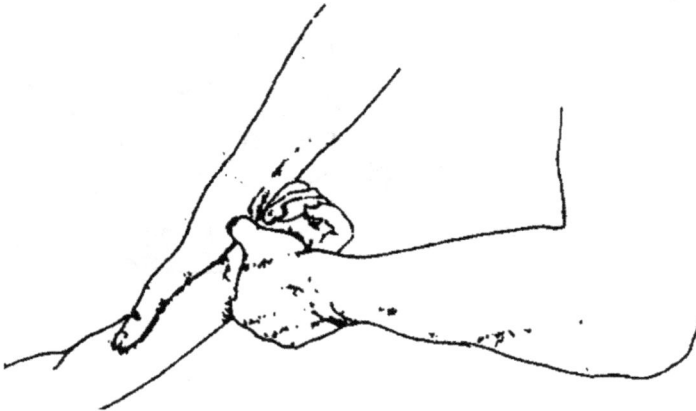

I-33

PETRISSAGING THE FOREARM.

Upper Arm Massage

- Bend your partner's elbow slightly, and let your subjects palm lay on his or her stomach. Decrease your height by spreading your legs apart so you don't need to bend as much and risk injury to your own back.

- Place your hands on top of your partner's upper arm and petrissage (knead) the muscles by passing the tissue from one hand to the other. Unlike the petrissage you did before, you have both of your hands free now. Be careful not to pinch.

- Perform this stroke about four times. Effleurage the entire arm with three repetitions.

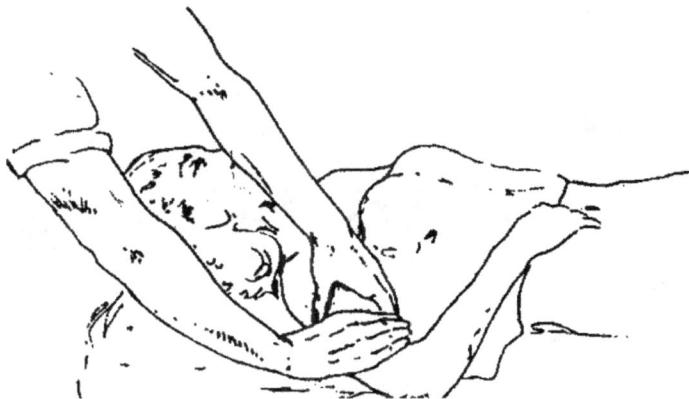

I-34

PETRISSAGE OVER THE UPPER ARM.

Shoulder Massage

The next massage addresses the shoulders.

- Place your hands (palms open), one on top of the shoulder and the other on the bottom of your partner's shoulder, (like a sandwich).

- Squeeze the shoulder with your palms and glide your palms in the opposite direction, back and forth, back and forth. This stroke feels wonderful.

- Repeat this stroke about four times. Once you are finished with the shoulder, effleurage the entire arm for a three repetitions, from the wrist to the shoulder again.

Note: You will notice we use effleurage in between every stroke. This is because it has such a soothing and calming effect on the receiver.

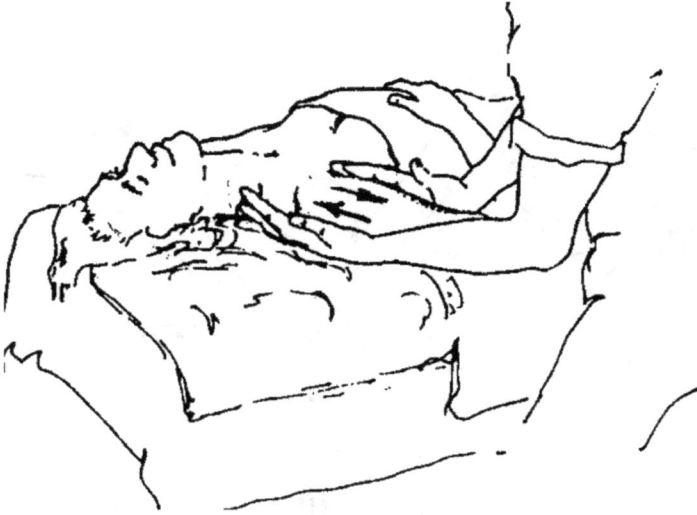

I-35

**SQUEEZE AND STROKE THE UPPER
SHOULDER IN OPPOSITE DIRECTIONS.**

Arm Stretch

- Raise the arm backward if possible (180 degrees). Perform this gently, paying close attention to any sign of discomfort displayed by your partner. Stop the stretching at the first sign of pain.

- If possible, hold the arm in this backward position for about thirty seconds.

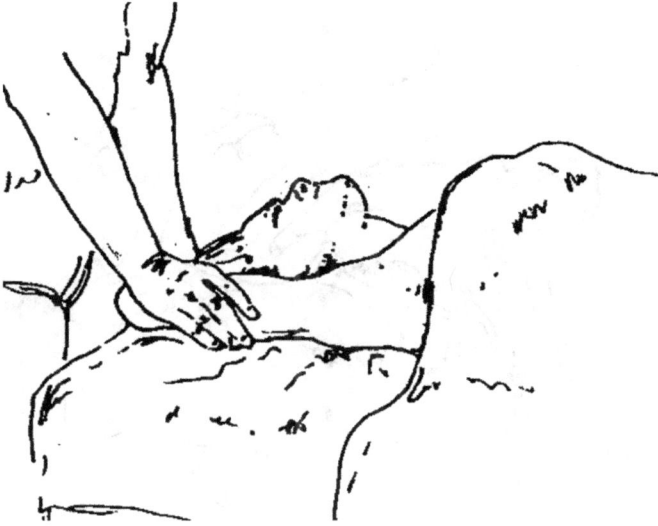

I-36

STRETCH THE ARM BACKWARD AND HOLD FOR ABOUT THIRTY SECONDS.

Massaging the Shoulder Blades

- Raise the arm slightly from the stretching position that you just completed. Support the arm with one of your hands.

- Now, place your other hand by your partner's elbow and stroke the upper arm (from the back side), passing the shoulder and the shoulder blade, then returning gently to the elbow. When passing your hand under the shoulder you need to elevate your partner slightly.

- Continue this stroke for three repetitions. See figures I-37 and I-38.

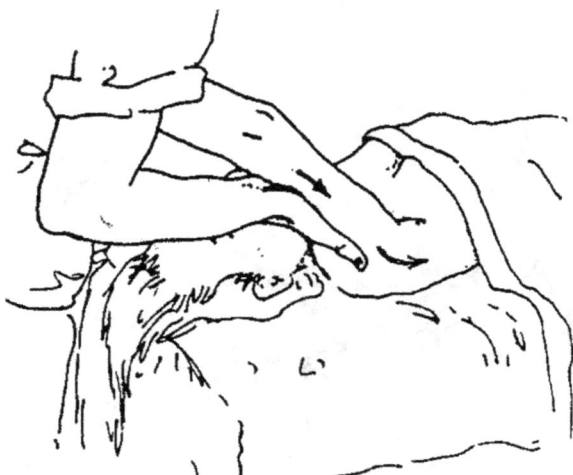

I-37

SUPPORT YOUR PARTNER'S ARM WITH ONE OF YOUR HANDS. WITH THE OTHER HAND, APPLY PRESSURE AND EFFLEURAGE THE UPPER ARM, PASSING THE SHOULDER AND THE SHOULDER BLADE.

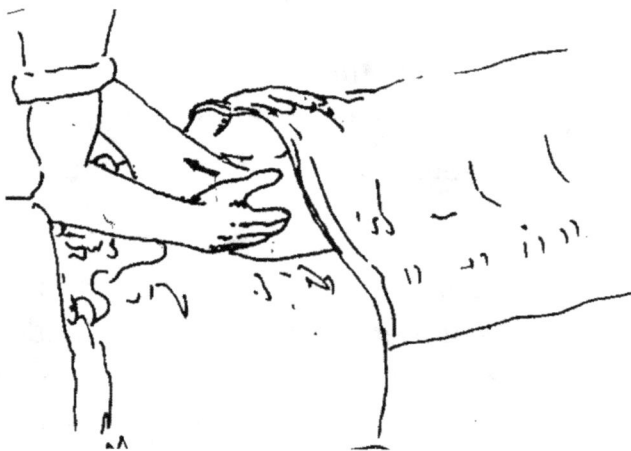

I-38

ON THE WAY BACK RELEASE SOME OF THE PRESSURE AND GLIDE BACK TOWARD YOUR STARTING POSITION BY THE ELBOW.

Nerve Strokes

Remember that you are in control. When you finish massaging the arm, place it back on the massage table at its original position. You control the situation now. Expect no help from your partner during massage, except once when you need your subject to turn over.

To complete the massage on this body part, use nerve strokes. Nerve strokes are light touches. This can be done with both of your hands barely touching the skin and hair follicles of the body part you just finished massaging. This stroke is pleasant, soothing, and pampering.

Leg Massage

Just as when we did arm massage, it's a good idea to use the body mechanics technique when doing leg massage, as it is a long stretch.

- Apply oil to your hands and spread it over the leg with effleurage strokes. This stroke starts at the foot and it ends by the waistline.

Note: Use discretion when massaging so close to the genital area; it may be arousing to your partner, to you, or to both. If you continue massaging this area, it may turn to something other than massage. As a massage therapist, you are warned over and over again that you may get into trouble if you get too intimate. You may lose your license or even be sued. Having said that, if you are already close with the person on the table, it may enhance the intimacy between the two of you even more. The only drawback in this case is that you may be tempted not to finish your massage...

- Use pressure on your way up to the hip area.

- On the way back to the feet, loosen up on the pressure and glide gently till reaching the foot again. Repeat this stroke three times.

Note: Remember that one of the purposes of effleurage is to evaluate your partner's condition. If you notice swelling, redness, bruises, rashes, or any other irregular signs, bring it to your partner's attention. Your partner will notice you are paying extra attention and will thank you.

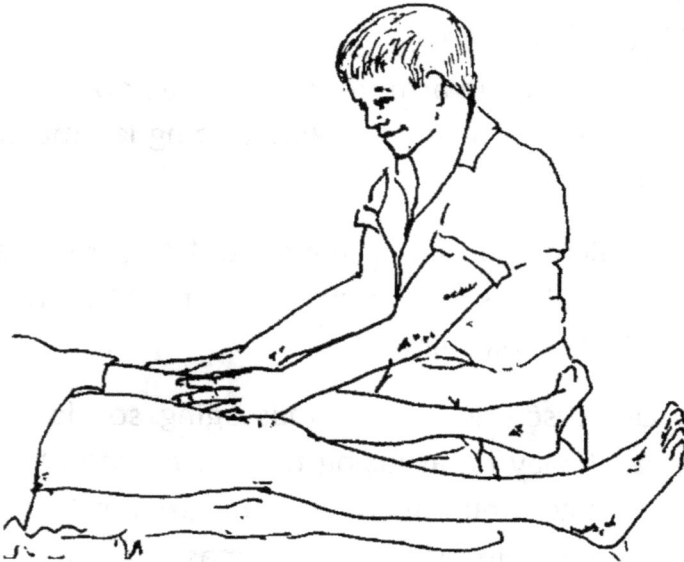

I-39

EFFLEURAGE STROKE OVER THE LEG.

Leg Petrissage

- Petrissage the entire leg, from the ankle all the way to the hip area. One repetition of petrissage is enough.

- Once you finish this stroke, effleurage the leg again for three repetitions. When performing this stroke, place your feet about two feet apart to decrease your height and to protect your back.

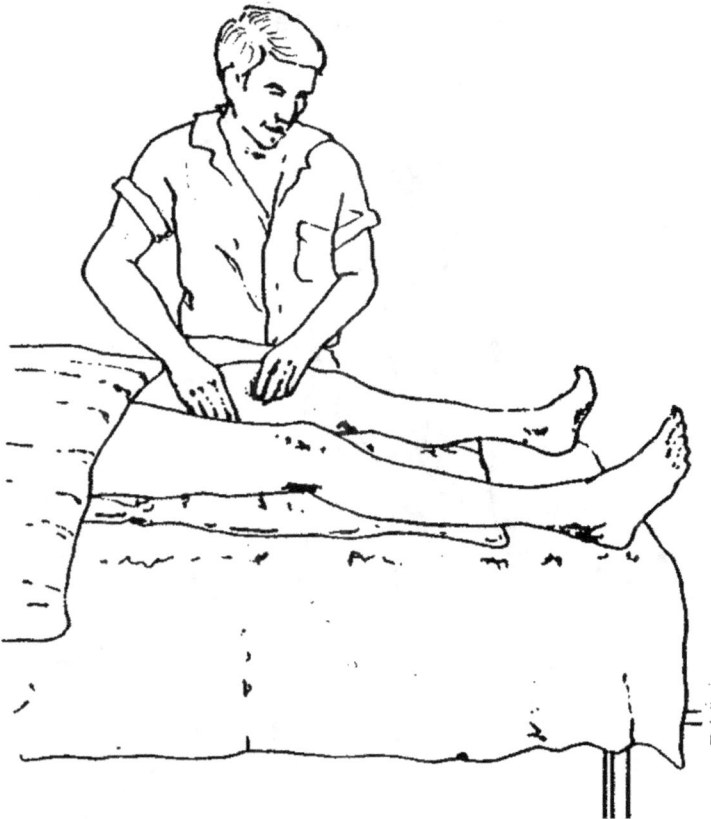

I-40

PETRISSAGE THE LEG (KNEADING) BY PASSING THE MUSCLE TISSUE FROM ONE HAND TO THE OTHER.

Compression over the Upper Leg Muscles

- Place both of your palms on top of the thigh, just above the knee.

- Lean into the stroke to achieve more pressure, and compress the tissue downward.

- Lift your hands and compress again in a different spot, until you have covered the entire upper leg. Don't forget to ask your partner if the pressure is too strong.

- Effleurage the entire leg three times.

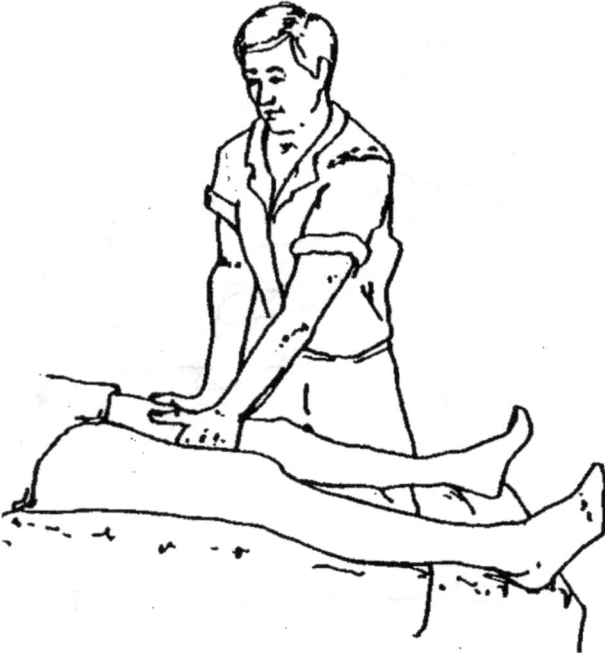

I-41

COMPRESSION OVER THE UPPER LEG MUSCLES.

Deep Effleurage over the Upper Leg

- Point your stiff fingers on both sides of the ankle.

- Apply pressure and glide with your finger tips up to the knee.

- Repeat this stroke three times and do the same to the upper leg, from the knee to the hip. Finish the leg massage by doing three repetitions of effleurage over the whole leg, as well as nerve strokes.

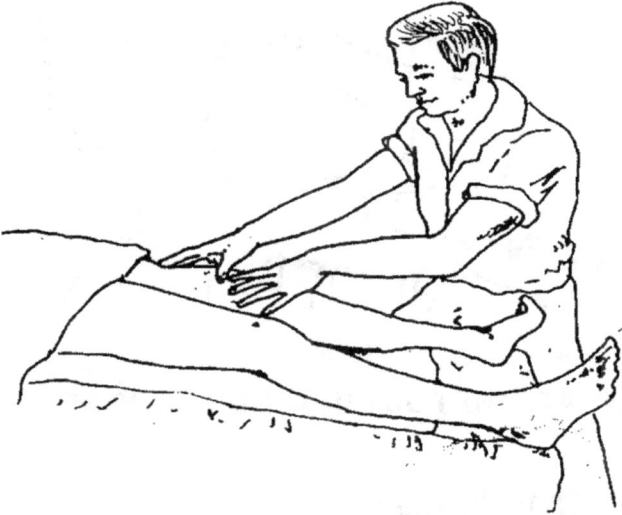

I-42

DEEP EFFLEURAGE STROKE IS DONE WITH FINGER TIPS.

Foot Rotations

- Raise the foot slightly from the table. Support the ankle with one of your hands and with your other hand support the foot by the toes.

- Rotate the foot in all directions forward, backward, left, and right. The rotation movement will help loosen the ankle joint.

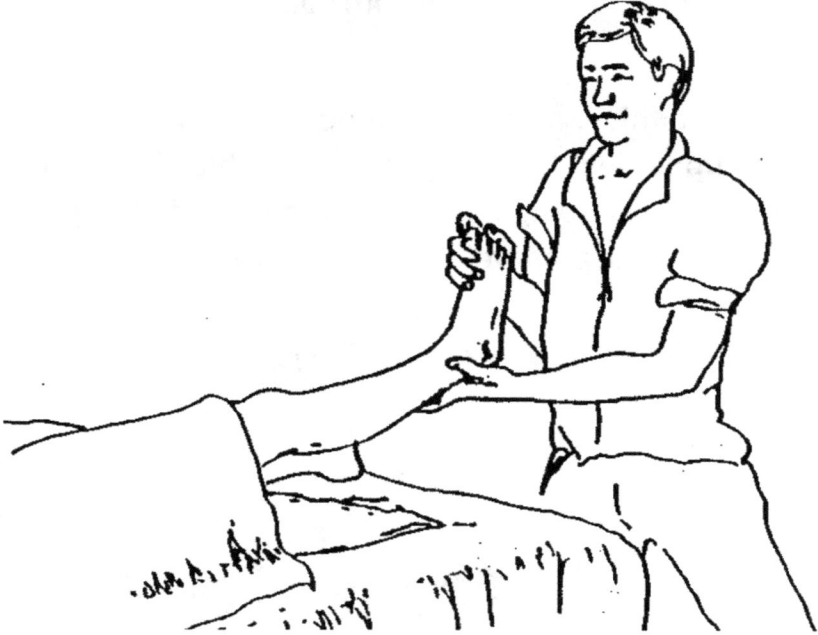

I-43

ROTATE THE FOOT IN ALL DIRECTIONS.

Bottom of the Foot Massage

- Lower your partner's leg onto the table.

- Hold your partner's toes with one hand. With the other hand make a fist.

- Press your fist close to your partner's toes and stroke with your knuckles the entire surface of the bottom of the foot. Repeat this stroke four times.

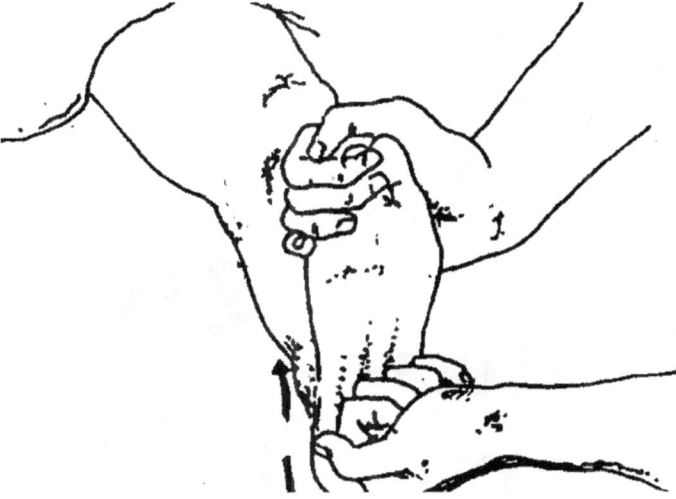

I-44

"THE AGONY OF THE FEET"

The feet are known to be the most neglected parts of our body. We rarely see the bottom of our feet, and they take a lot of punishment through our lifetime. Treat them well when giving massage. Some people like foot massage so much that they willing to pay a lot of money for a professional foot massage. This kind of massage is known as reflexology massage.

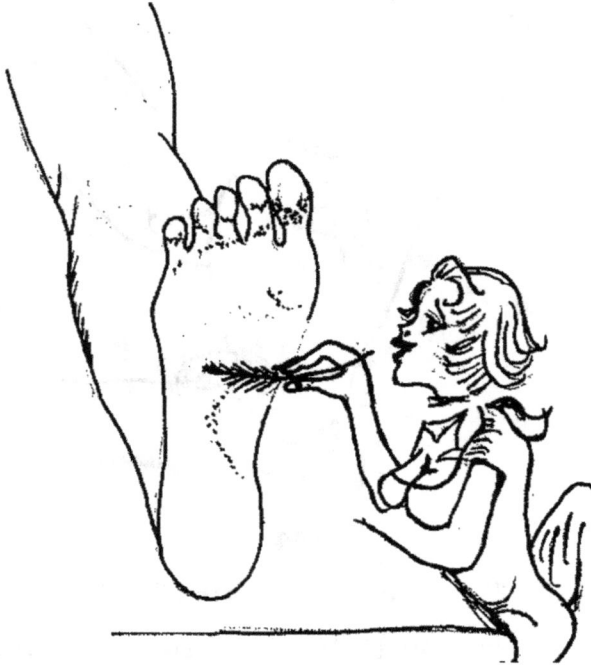

I-45

REFLEXOLOGY (FOOT MASSAGE) IS NO TICKLE MATTER.

- Use your thumbs stroking the bottom of the feet, one thumb following another.

- Apply pressure with your thumbs and stroke the entire foot.

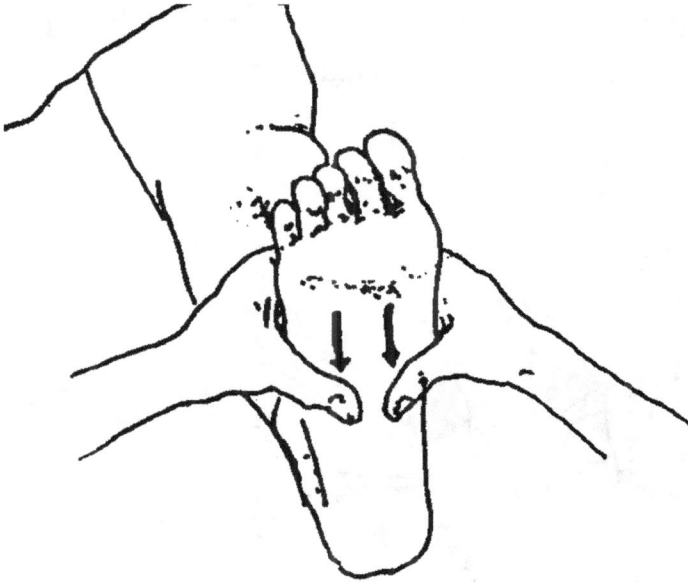

I-46

**USE YOUR THUMBS TO MASSAGE EVERY
SQUARE INCH OF THE BOTTOM OF THE FEET.**

Top of the Foot Massage

- Now massage the top of the foot, the part you see when standing up. As discussed earlier, massage only the soft tissue between the bones, but not the bones themselves.

- The next stroke is done with the thumbs as well. Starting between the toes, apply pressure with your thumbs, one following the other, and glide all the way toward the connection of the foot with the leg.

- Do the same to the soft tissue of the whole upper foot. One repetition should be sufficient.

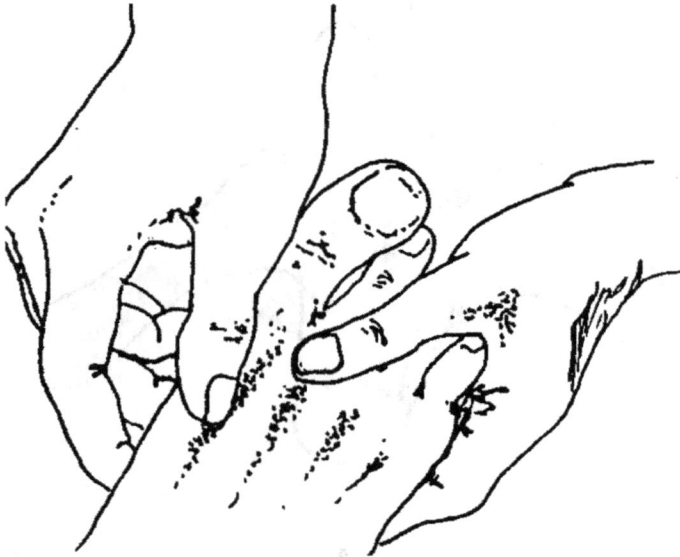

I-47

USE FRICTION STROKES ON THE SOFT TISSUE IN BETWEEN THE BONY AREA.

Toes Massage

- Take each toe between your thumb and index finger.

- "Milk" it (pull and glide gently from the root of the toe to the tip, let go and start again). Repeat two or three times on each toe).

- Give the nail area a squeeze as you finish massaging each toe.

- Stroke the area between the toes a couple of times. Use your thumb and index finger in a milking motion.

Getting a good foot massage can be a real treat; it may even give your partner a "high." A good foot massage is known to contribute to the relaxing and surrendering of the body. You have to feel it yourself to know what I mean.

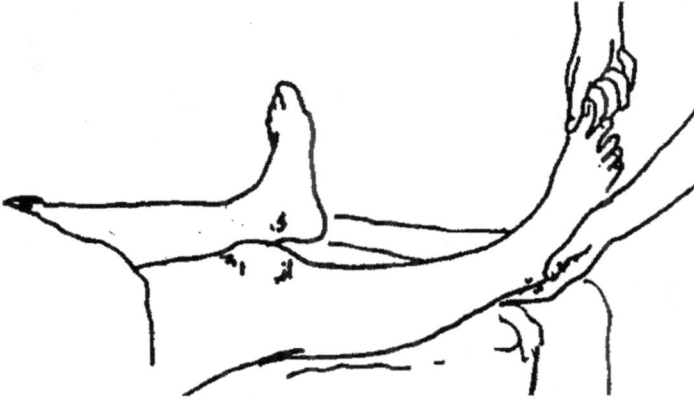

1-48

TAKE EACH TOE BETWEEN YOUR THUMB AND INDEX FINGER AND "MILK" IT A FEW TIMES.

- Effleurage the whole leg three times and finish the leg massage with nerve strokes, very light and calming touches. Pass your fingers over the leg lightly, barely touching the skin and the hair follicles.

- Once you complete one leg, repeat the same strokes on the other leg.

After you have finished, ask your partner to turn over to the other side (on his or her stomach). Hold the cover in a way that your partner may be able to turn without losing his or her dignity. By now your partner can't help seeing how dependable you are. Your subject has developed a sense of security and trust in you, not to be taken lightly.

CHAPTER - 3
Massage—Facing Down

If you remember, you have just finished working on the legs. In the previous chapter, we described massage of the front side of the legs. Now you have turned your partner over (facing down), and you are going to continue massaging the legs, this time from the back side.

When doing the back of the legs, ask your partner's permission to do the buttocks as well, because this area contains a lot of muscles and nerves. One of them is well known as the sciatic nerve. When the sciatic nerve is pinched, it radiates a tremendous amount of pain to the buttocks and legs. Sometimes it is so severe that the pain or numbness can extend all the way down to the feet. People suffering from lower back pain often have a pinched sciatic nerve.

The Sciatic Nerve Extension
The sciatic nerve originates in the lower back, and it extends all the way to our feet. It is as thick as our thumb in some areas. Lower back pain can often be the cause of numbness and pain traveling all the way down to the feet.

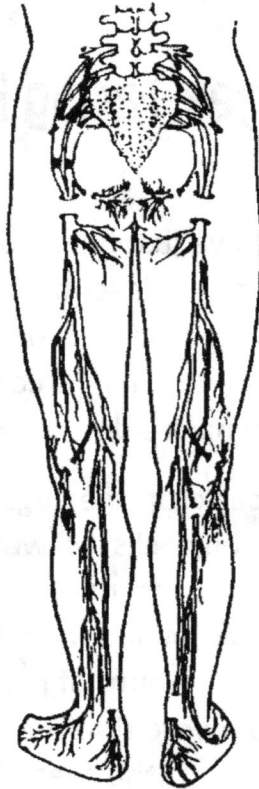

I-49

A VIEW OF THE SCIATIC NERVE.

Back of the Leg Massage

- As always, start by applying oil to your hands and spread it evenly to the back of the leg with effleurage strokes, from the ankle all the way up passed the buttocks.

- Make three repetitions.

Remember to practise your body mechanics technique here...It's a long stretch.

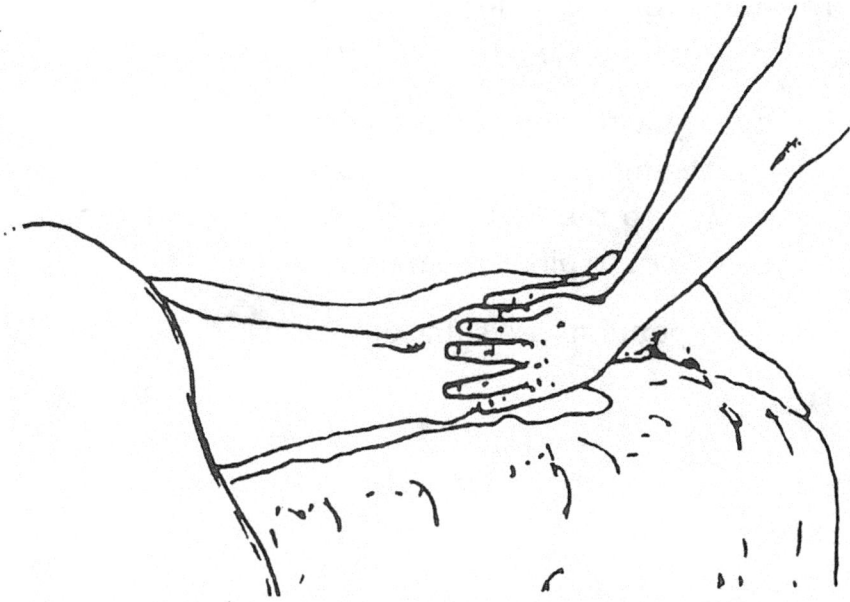

I-50

EFFLEURAGE STROKES, OVER THE LOWER PORTION OF THE LEG.

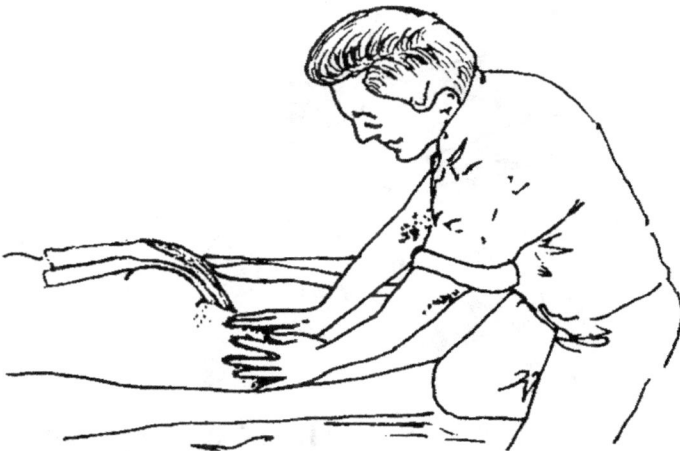

I-51

BACK OF THE LEG EFFLEURAGE, OVER THE FLOOR.

The next stroke over the back of the leg is petrissage. Start by your partner's ankle.

- Squeeze with your palms against the calf muscles and pass the muscle tissue from one hand to the other all the way to the buttocks. When doing petrissage, be careful not to pinch the muscles.

- Two repetitions are sufficient.

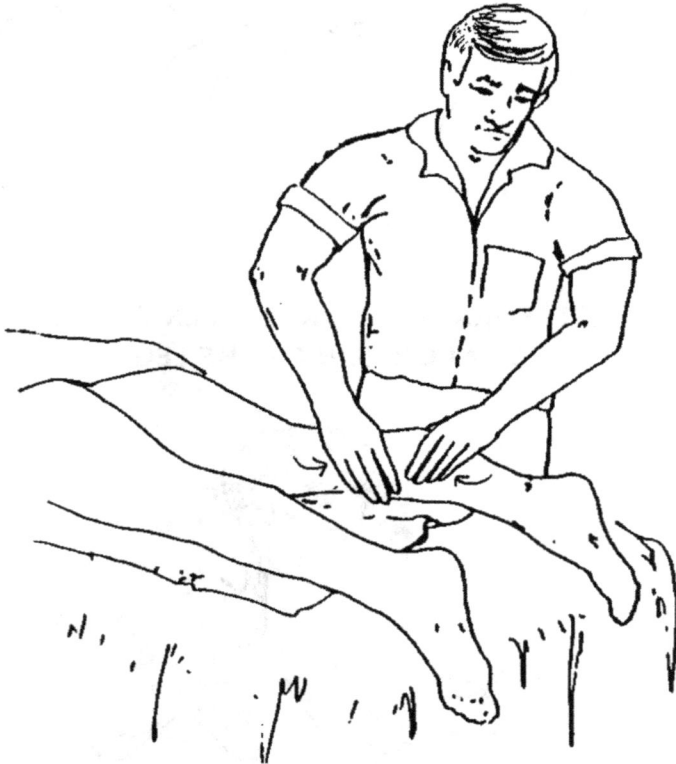

I-52

PETRISSAGE STROKES OVER THE LOWER LEG MUSCLES.

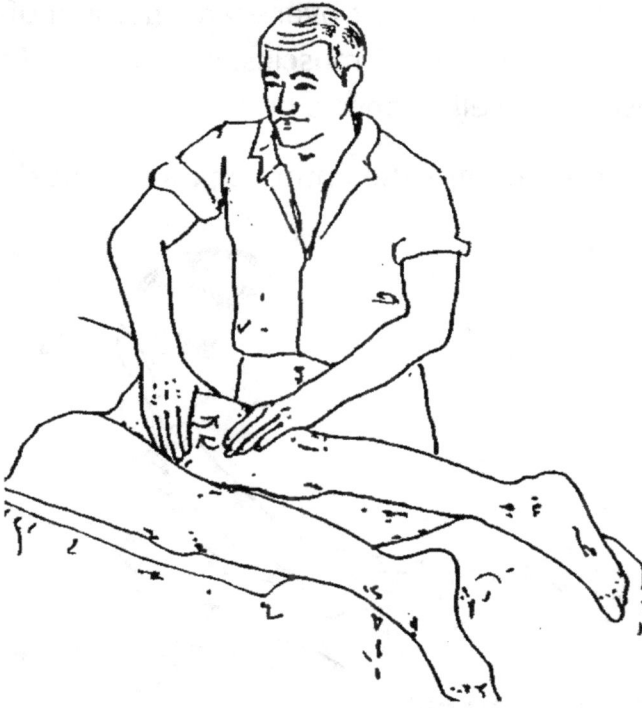

I -53

PETRISSAGE STROKES OVER THE UPPER LEG.

- Once you're done petrissaging the lower and the upper leg, follow up with three repetitions of effleurage on the entire leg.

Deep Penetration

If you want to reach into the deeper muscles, use deep effleurage.

- Stiffen your finger then dig into the leg muscles and glide, one hand following another for about three repetitions.

- Use these deep strokes over a large number of muscles, such as over the calf muscles, on the top of the thigh muscles as well as on the buttocks.

- Finally, effleurage the entire leg three times.

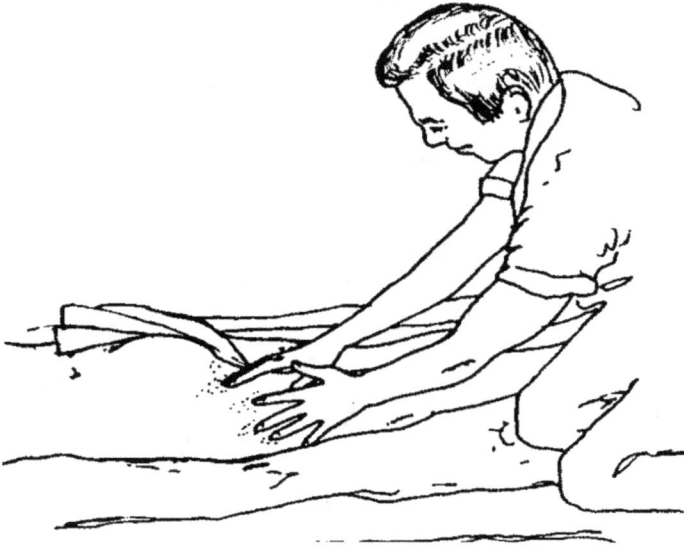

I-54

DEEP EFFLEURAGE. PRESS YOUR FINGERTIPS AGAINST THE MUSCLE TISSUE AND GLIDE.

Friction

To use friction on the legs, compress and move the underlying tissue. Use your thumbs by sinking them into the tissue and moving them in left and right directions, as shown in the next illustration. Friction has a tendency to penetrate deep. It breaks adhesions and gives relief to the deep muscles that otherwise can't be reached with superficial strokes.

Friction is best to use over the legs, buttocks, and over spasm areas. Effleurage the entire leg three more times.

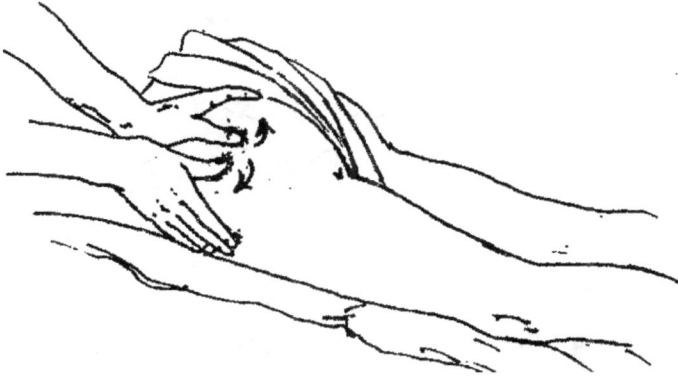

I-55

FRICTION: PRESS YOUR THUMBS DEEP INTO THE MUSCLE TISSUE AND STROKE LEFT AND RIGHT.

Leg Stretch

Stretching is an important action, not only for flexibility, but also for achieving an important state of relaxation. Try to combine stretching with your massage routine whenever possible.

- Bend the leg until resistance is felt. Ask your partner for feedback regarding any discomfort.

- Once the maximum possible stretch has been achieved, hold for thirty seconds, then lower the leg gently back to its original position.

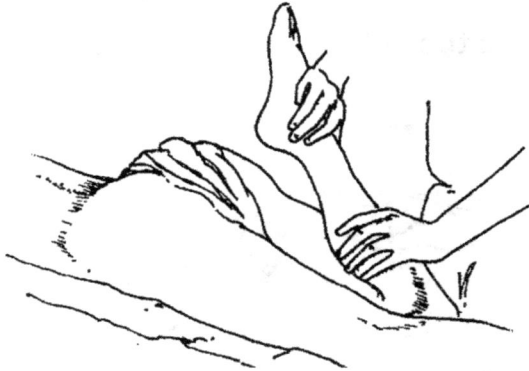

I-56

STRETCH THE LEG AND HOLD BACKWARD FOR ABOUT THIRTY SECONDS.

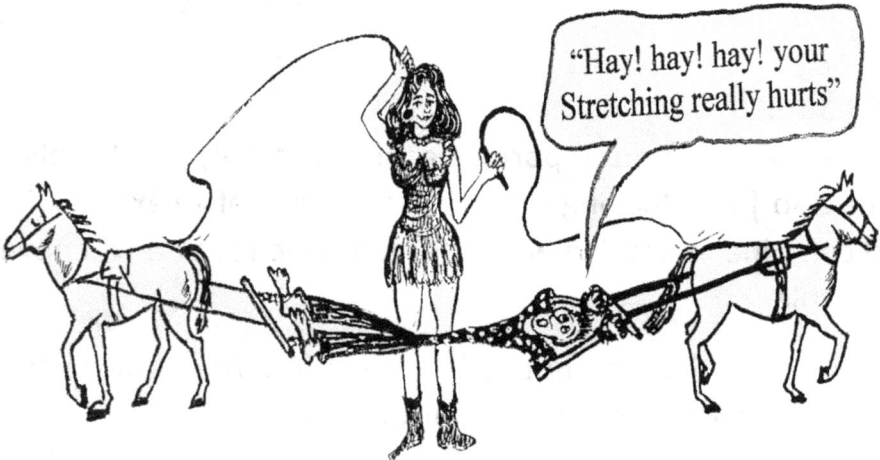

"Hay! hay! hay! your Stretching really hurts"

I-57

STRETCHING CAN BE GOOD FOR YOU.

- Effleurage the leg three times and finish with gentle and relaxing nerve strokes all over the leg.

At this point you have completed massaging one leg. Move to the other side and massage the other leg in the same way.

Back Pain

Before we start talking about how to massage the back, I want to devote a few words to back pain, as so many of us fall into that category.

Back pain strikes 90 percent of all Americans, and there are very few permanent solutions to this common problem. Your partner may be one of those people who suffers from back pain. If this is the case, he or she may be in luck as you may be able to ease that pain by giving your partner a back massage.

Back pain does not heal itself if left untreated. Once the back is injured, it will remain vulnerable. All it takes is a little bend or back twist to trigger the pain again.

Back massage and stretching are very effective and drug free methods which can ease that pain.

There are two major areas of back pain. The upper back and the lower back. Upper back pain can be felt usually between the shoulders. It can give signals of pain to the head, neck, and shoulders, as well as to the arms.

Lower back pain, on the other hand, cases pain in the buttocks, in the legs and feet, Common side effects are stiffness, acute pain, difficulty walking, bending, going to the bathroom, and so on.

You can throw your back out of balance in a variety of ways. One common way is through impact caused by a car accident. Sometimes it is a result of heavy lifting, lifting the wrong way, herniated disc, spinal stenosis, rheumatoid arthritis, sciatica, straining a pinched nerve, a sports injury, excess weight, pregnancy, walking with high heels and more. Back pain can be downright nasty and disabling. You may feel like an old person. You have a decrease in range of motion; after an injury you may start to watch every move you make in order not to aggravate you back. You may feel extreme pain, stiffness, and difficulty doing the simplest things you once took for granted. You may start to feel sorry for yourself, and depression can follow.

Back Massage

If you know how to give a good back massage, people may be drawn to you. Try devoting more time massaging the back. If you notice a painful area, try loosening the area around the painful spot first, then work your way to the center of the pain. You will obtain better results that way. When someone is in a lot of pain, always start gently, then increase pressure as you loosen the painful area. Although all your massage is important, your partner will remember you for the back massage more then anything else. Even if you are unsure of your massage skills yet, concentrate and do your best with back massage.

Back Effleurage

- Stand behind your partner's head, apply oil to your hands, and use (you guessed it) effleurage strokes to spread the massage oil evenly across your partner's back, neck, and shoulders.

- Apply pressure with your palms and effleurage the whole back three times.

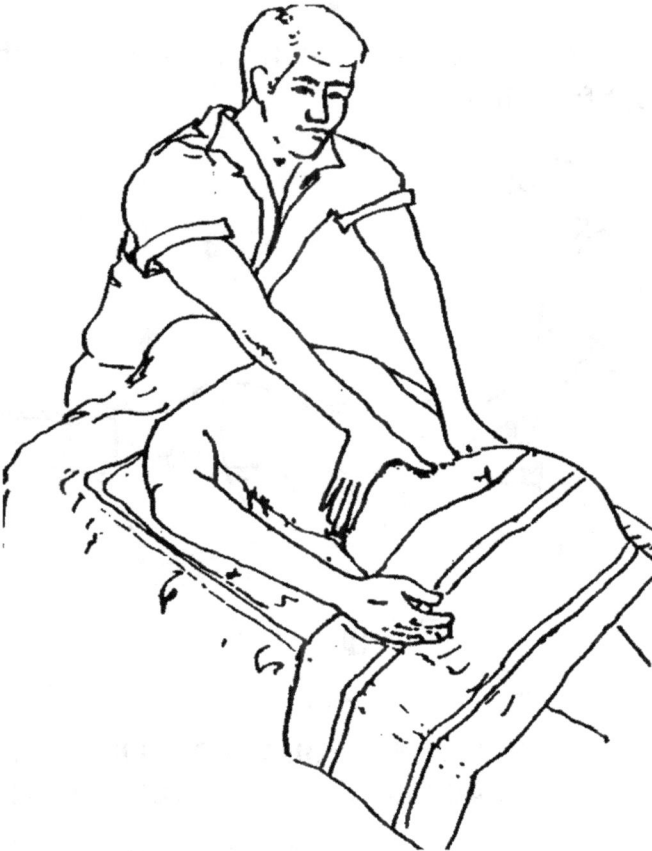

I-58

EFFLEURAGE THE ENTIRE BACK WITH SLOW MOTIONS AND USE YOUR WEIGHT TO DELIVER PRESSURE.

Neck and Back Massage

- Make a fist with each of your palms and place them on the shoulders close to the neck.

- Apply pressure to your strokes using your body weight as leverage.

- Twist your fists with pressure left and right, left and right.

- Massage the area between the neck and the shoulders about four times.

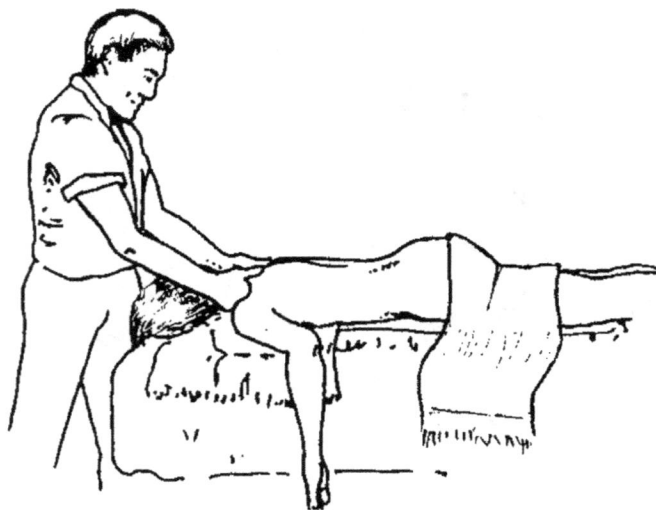

I-59

PRESS YOUR FIST AGAINST YOUR PARTNER'S SHOULDER AND TWIST BACK AND FORTH SEVERAL TIMES.

- Keep pressure on your partner's upper shoulders and without releasing the pressure on the shoulders, start opening your fist slowly as you glide the heel of your hands (the pinky side) on both sides of the spine all the way down to the buttocks. This tends to stretch the tight muscles on both sides of the spine and subsequently releases tension from the back.

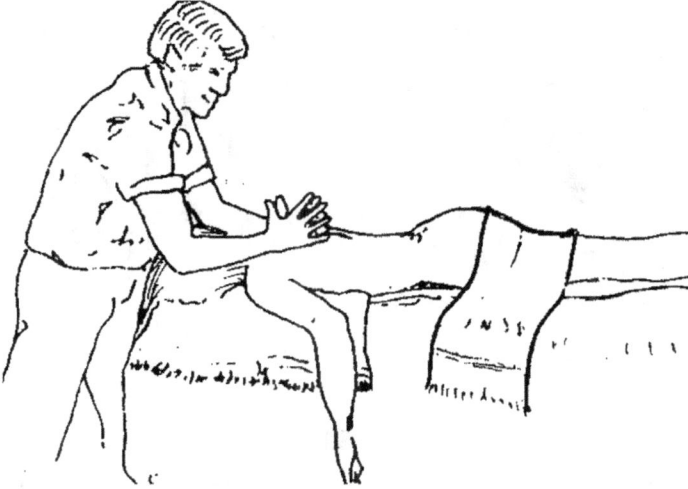

I-60

OPEN YOUR FIST SLOWLY AND GLIDE GENTLY ON BOTH SIDES OF THE SPINE.

- Release the pressure and glide lightly back to the neck and shoulders - your starting position.

- Make a fist again close to the neck and shoulders.

- Massage the shoulders with your fists the same way, then open your fist and repeat the gliding motion on both sides of the spine.

- Do these strokes three times and follow with effleurage on the entire back.

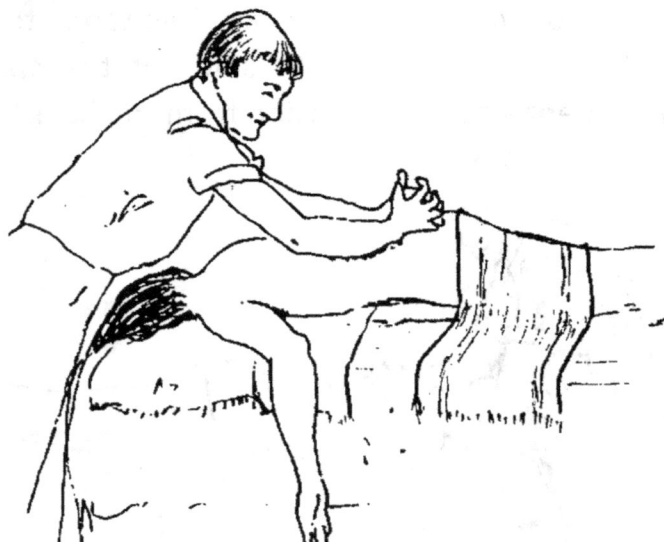

I-61

**CONTINUE GLIDING WITH THAT STROKE ALL
THE WAY TO THE BUTTOCKS.**

Treatment for a Knotted Back

The shoulders blades, (the large flat triangular bones that lie against the ribs in the upper back, also known as the scapula) and the upper back in general are common areas for accumulation of knotted muscles caused by bad posture and a stressful lifestyle. As you are stroking the back, you will sometimes notice these knots in the underlying tissue. They will probably feel like little hard balls—tangled and lumpy. When pressing on them, they are going to hurt a little, but after working on them for a while, they will get smoother and feel better. Those lumps are known as knots because they have the shape and hardness of a knot. You will notice them especially surrounding the shoulder blade and upper shoulders.

To treat these tangled muscles, press your thumb directly on top of them and sustain a pressure for about ten or fifteen seconds, then release and go to the next knotted muscle. Another way is to use friction strokes. Depress your thumbs into the knotted area and move your thumbs left, right, left, right (friction mode) to work out the underlying tissue. Don't forget to get feedback from your partner by asking, "How does it feel?" or "Am I being too hard on you?" or maybe "Would you like me to lighten up?" and so on.

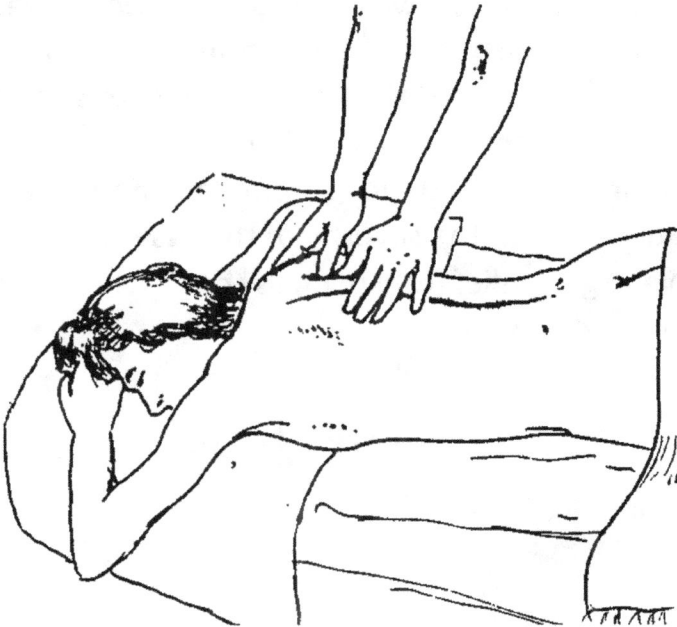

I-62

USE FRICTION WITH YOUR THUMBS OVER THE KNOTTED AREA SUCH AS AROUND THE SHOULDER BLADE.

Neck Stretching

- Stand behind your partner's head.

- Place your fingers by the hair line in the back of the neck. You are going to notice the ridge of the skull.

- Place your fingers along that ridge and pull firmly toward you, (don't put pressure on the ears). Sustain that momentum for about thirty seconds. This technique, as well as pulling on the feet, will cause the spine to stretch. As a direct result, the spaces between the vertebras and between the discs will enlarge and may give relief to pinched nerves. Once you accomplish that, there is going to be less pressure on the nerves, and the pain will start to subside. This is a major accomplishment for a back-pain sufferer. You may need to do several of these treatments (it depends on the severity of the case) but you will be able to give relief from pain, as I have seen it happening over and over and again.

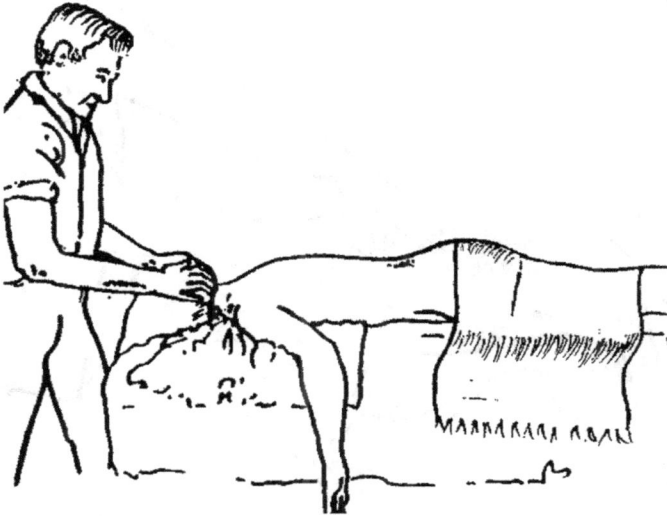

I-63

PRESS WITH YOUR FINGERS AT THE BASE OF THE SKULL. PULL AND HOLD FOR THIRTY SECONDS.

Massaging around the Shoulder Blade

- Move to your partner's side where his arm is resting. You will notice a large flat bone on each side of the shoulders where the arms connect to the body. That bone is the shoulder blade (or scapula).

- Use deep effleurage strokes around that bone with stiff fingers just to loosen up the area first..

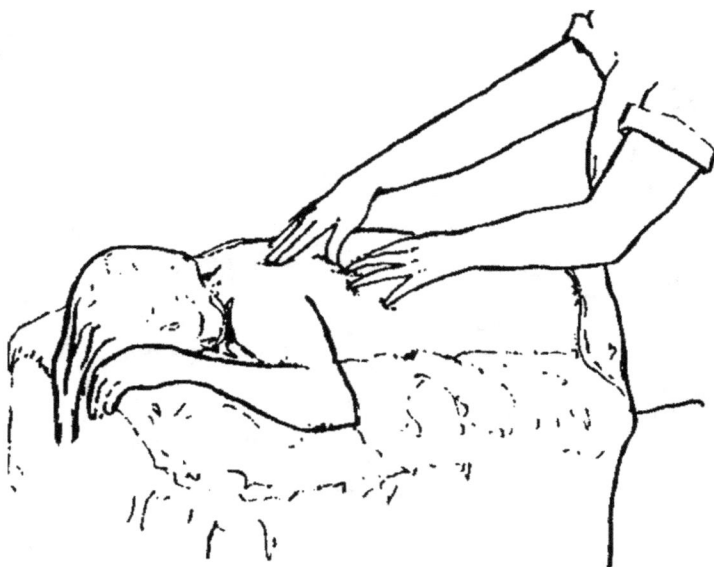

I-64

PRESS YOUR STIFF FINGERS AND GLIDE WITH PRESSURE ALL AROUND THE SHOULDER BLADE.

As mentioned above, the shoulder blade area has a tendency to accumulate knots (lumpy, tangled muscles). If knots are detected, be patient. Use friction strokes followed with effleurage strokes. Eventually these knots will subside and so will the pain.

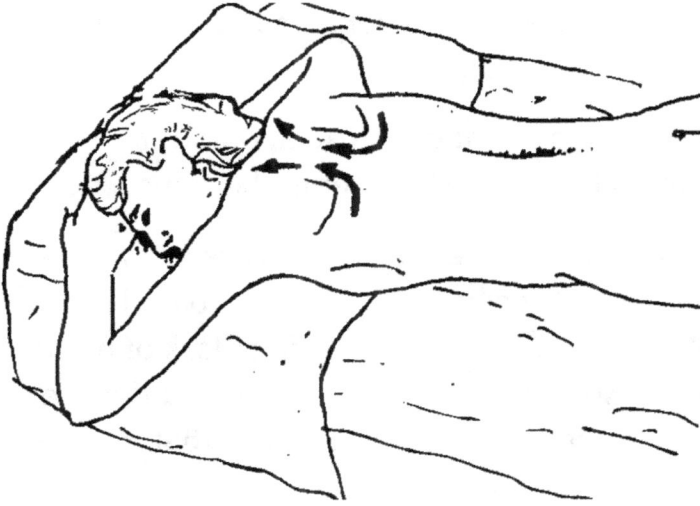

I-65

STROKES DIRECTION AROUND THE SHOULDER BLADE.

- Continue with effleurage all over the entire back for three repetitions.

- Try locating the ribs and work between them inside the soft tissue, using long strokes of effleurage and stiff fingers.

Shoulder Blade, Vibrations

Sometimes a shoulder can be so uptight that we easily notice a definite decrease in its mobility. This is known as a "frozen shoulder." If this has happened to your friend or spouse, you may be able to help by continuing to work on the shoulder blade using the vibration technique.

- Point your fingers right into the shoulder blade and make a fast, vibrating motion with them—right, left, right, left, with a general motion downward toward the middle back.

- Repeat the vibration stroke about four times, then you can do the other shoulder in the same way.

Note: In general, every kind of stroke or massage that we do on one side of the body, we have to do to the other side. If we don't, it will cause an imbalance or lack of harmony. Your partner will soon notice that the side you did the massage on is looser and lighter than the side that didn't receive a massage. If you are not sure about that, try giving a massage to someone on one hand and walk away. Most likely you will be asked, "What about the other hand?"

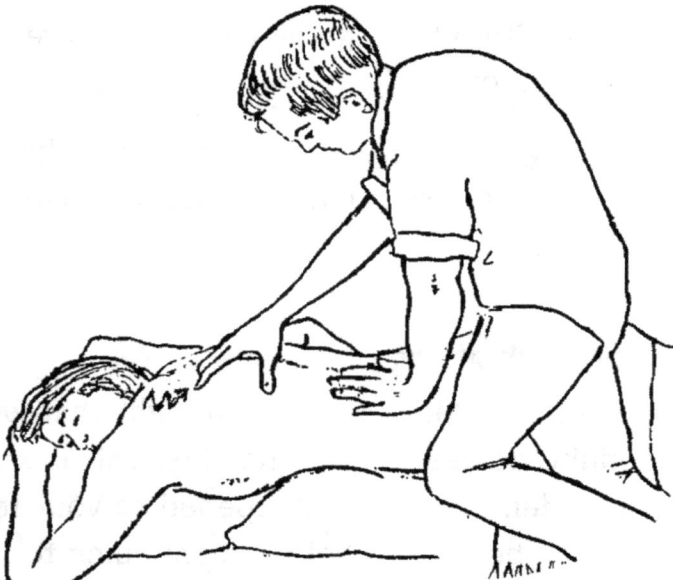

I-66

VIBRATION—PRESS YOUR FINGERS INTO THE MUSCLE TISSUE AND MAKE RAPID, VIBRATING MOTIONS.

Stretching the Shoulder Blade

- Gently lift the arm next to you, bend it at the elbow, and let it rest on the lower back. If you feel resistance or if your partner complains about being uncomfortable, skip this treatment and go on to your next stroke. Encourage your partner to tell you of any discomfort he or she may feel.

- With the palm resting on the lower back, notice that the shoulder blade is now protruding. Place your fingers under the shoulder blade and pull it upwards toward you, holding for fifteen seconds. This will cause the shoulder blade muscles to stretch and relax. Performing this stretch will not cause pain to your partner. It looks worse than it feels.

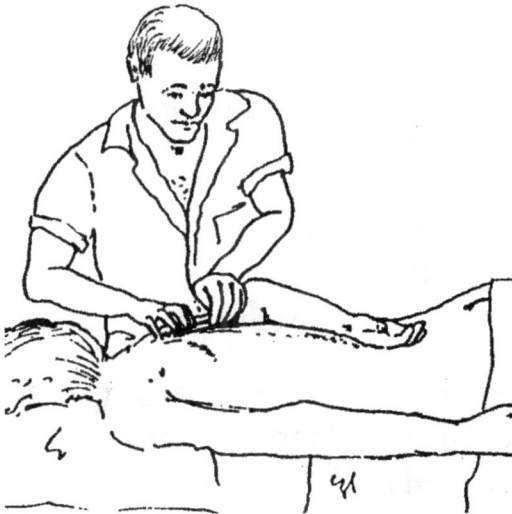

I-67

STRETCHING THE SHOULDER BLADE—PLACE YOUR FINGERTIPS UNDERNEATH THE SHOULDER BLADE AND PULL IT TOWARD YOU.

Massaging the inside of the Shoulder Blade

The inside the shoulder blade contains many muscles. Those muscles are responsible for keeping the arm attached to our body. Sometimes those muscles become irritated, as if they are practically begging for attention.

For the inside of the shoulder blade, friction strokes are the most effective.

- Press your thumbs into the shoulder blade muscle tissue.

- Glide them left and right until you have covered the entire inside of the shoulder blade.

For a visual demonstration, refer back to I-62.

Probing Into the Shoulder Muscles

The upper shoulders can become painful, especially if your partner works on a computer or has a desk job. Here is what you can do to help:

- Dig in with your thumb on the upper shoulder muscle, applying pressure and gliding with your thumb toward the neck. Do this slowly, from the tip of the shoulders to the neck.

- Repeat three times. Don't be afraid to exert some pressure. The shoulders can take lots of punishment. This is the kind of pain that feels good!

- Now that you are through working on one shoulder, practise the same massage strokes on the other shoulder.

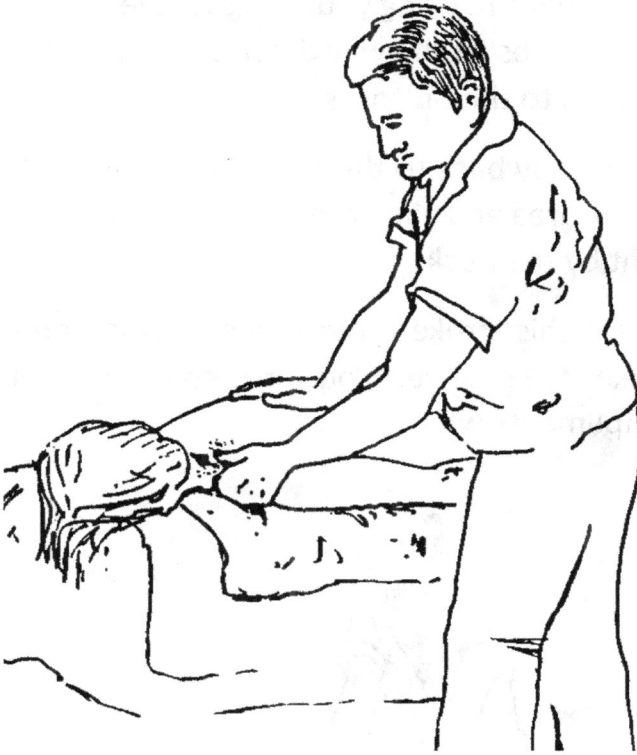

I-68

STROKE WITH YOUR THUMB WITH LOTS OF PRESSURE OVER THE UPPER SHOULDER TOWARD THE NECK.

Massaging the Area on Each Side of the Spine

Although we never directly massage the spine, since it is a bony area, we can massage the area along the side of the spine. This area extends from the neck all the way down to the buttocks.

- Stand behind your partner's head and press with your thumbs on both sides of the spine where the neck connects to the shoulders.

- Apply pressure using your weight as leverage and glide your thumbs all the way down the entire length of the spine up to the buttocks.

- On the way back to the neck, open your palms flat on the hip area and glide them gently to the same starting point by the neck.

- Repeat this stroke three times. This is an enjoyable stroke to receive. You are going to get lots of compliments when you use it.

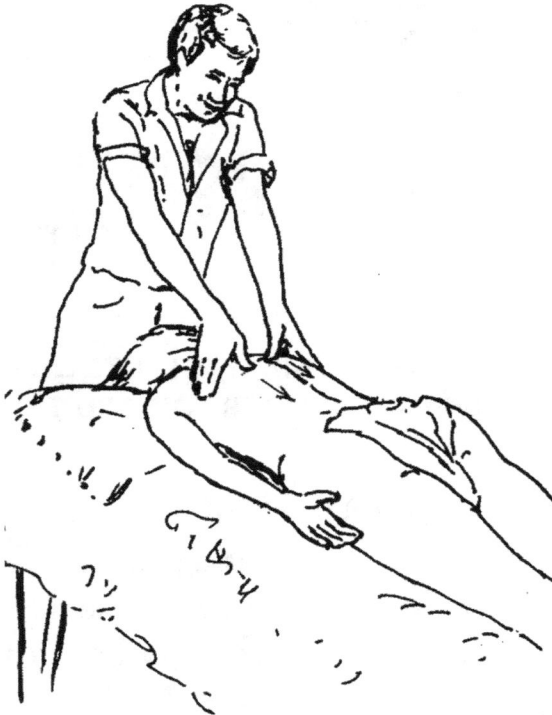

I-69

PRESS YOUR THUMBS ON BOTH SIDES OF THE SPINE AND GLIDE ALL THE WAY TO THE BUTTOCKS AREA.

Back Petrissage

- Stand beside your partner, close to one of his or her arms.

- Petrissage half of the back, starting with the part of the back that is farthest away from you.

- Start petrissaging from the upper shoulder, then continue petrissaging the rest of the back which is way from you all the way to the buttocks. Practice passing the skin and muscle tissue from one hand to the other. This stroke feels absolutely wonderful. Repeat it twice.

The next two illustrations will give you a better understanding of this stroke.

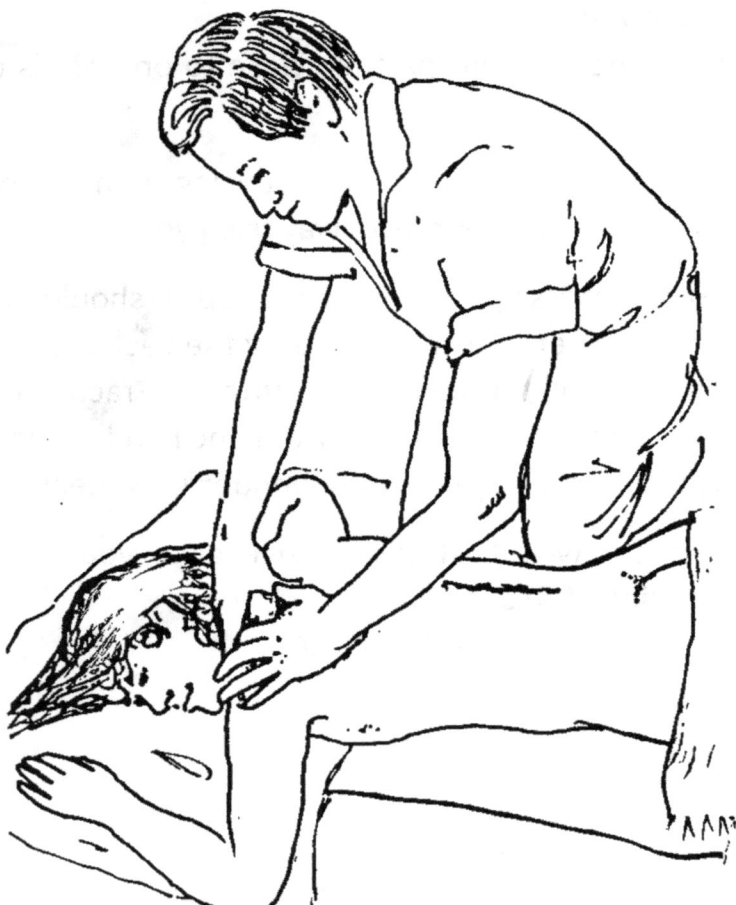

I-70

PETRISSAGING (ON THE FLOOR) ON THE SHOULDER AND THE BACK WHICH IS FARTHEST AWAY FROM YOU.

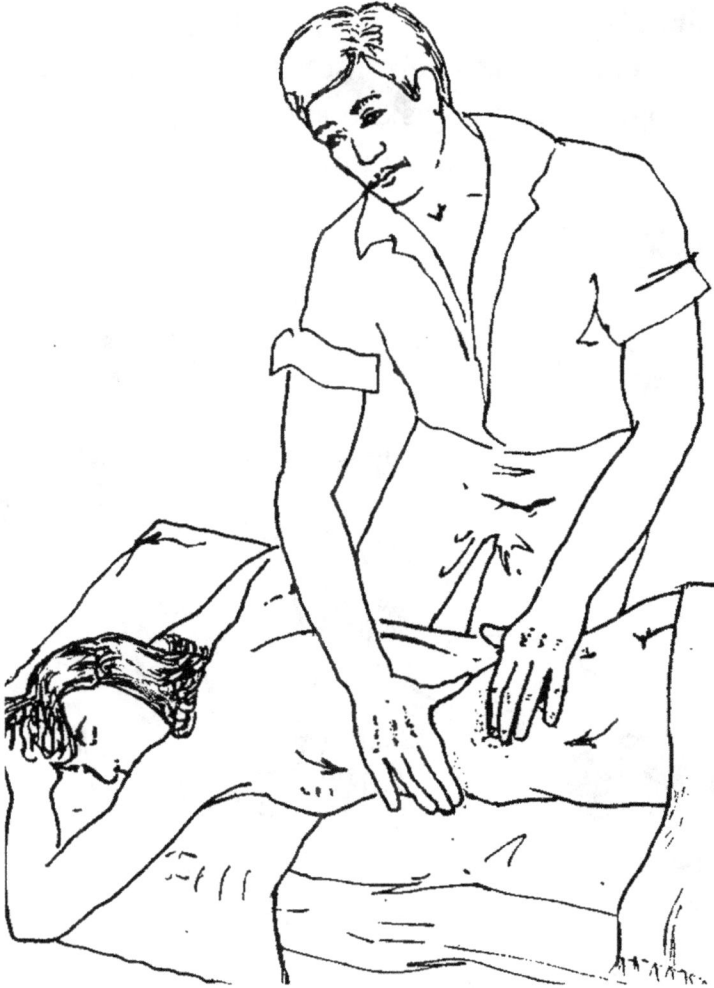

I-71

PETRISSAGING (ON THE TABLE) FROM THE SHOULDER ALL THE WAY TO THE BUTTOCKS.

Cross Fiber Strokes

Cross fiber strokes are sometimes referred to as crisscrossing. Those strokes are soothing and are perfect to use just prior to the end of your massage, (your grand finale).

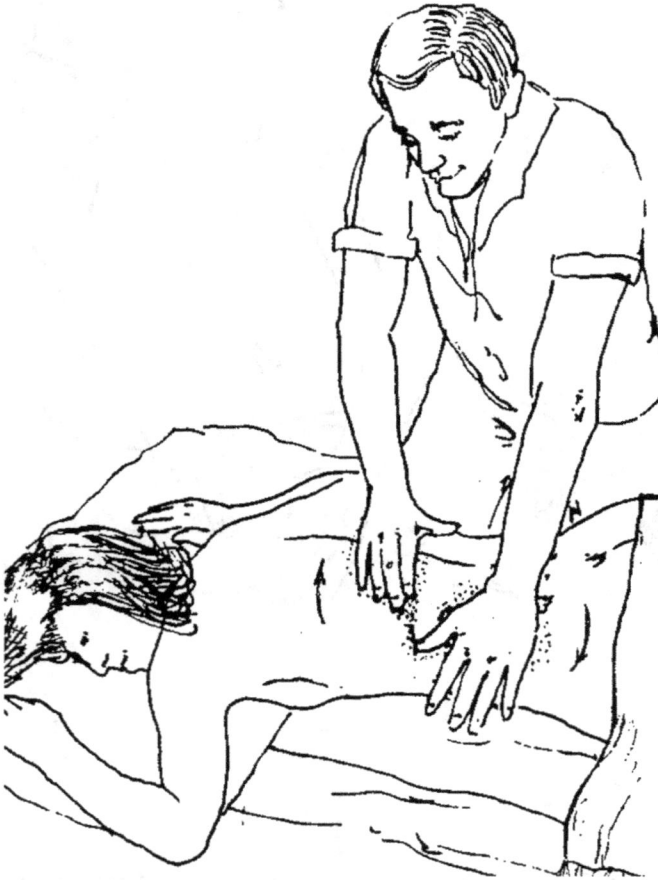

I-72

PRESS YOUR PALMS AGAINST THE BACK AND GLIDE THEM IN OPPOSITE DIRECTIONS.

Cross fiber means massaging against the direction of the muscle fibers. While doing cross fiber massage, you will be using effleurage strokes.

- Place your hands flat on your partner's back, close to the shoulder area. Press firmly and glide across the width of your partner's back in the opposite direction. In other words, one hand is moving forward while the other glides backward.

- Massage the whole back from the shoulders to the buttocks and from the buttocks back to the shoulders. Repeat this stroke about three times.

- Once finished, effleurage the back again for three repetitions. See I-58

- Go to the other side of your partner and do the same on that side using petrissage to do the other half of the back and follow with cross fiber strokes.

- Once done, go behind your partner's head and effleurage the entire back.

After working on your partner for as long as you have, he or she should be feeling relaxed and sedated, almost limp and sleepy. You are close to the end of your massage, so you don't want to agitate or over stimulate at this point.

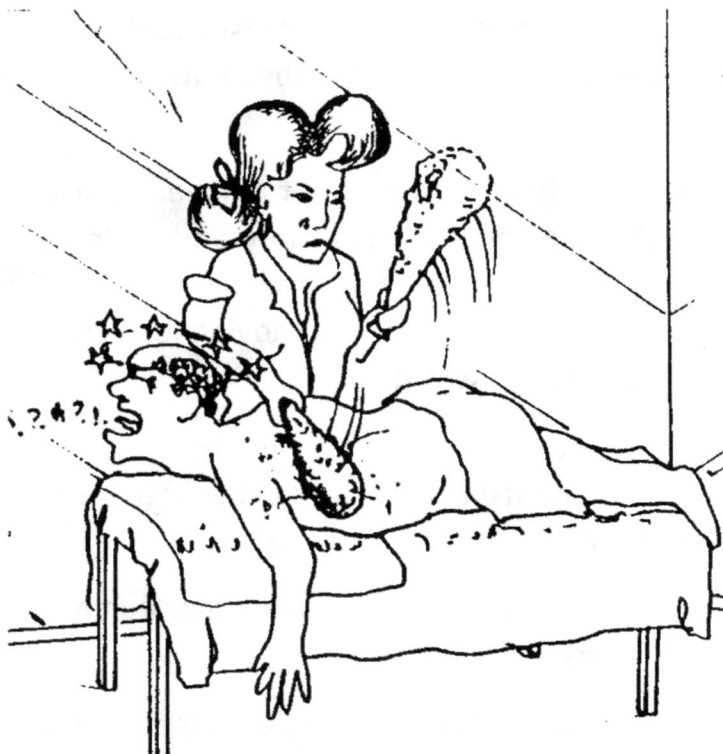

I-73

"I AM GOING TO GIVE YOU MASSAGE THAT YOU WILL *NEVER* FORGET."

Nerve Stroke over the Back

Very gently and barely touching the skin, perform that magic with your fingers. Touch briefly all over the back from the hips to the head. Try to cover every inch of the back area. Administer nerve strokes to the back for about three repetitions. Don't be surprised if goose bumps appear on the surface of the skin; it means your partner is experiencing a great sense of pleasure, thanks to you.

Reminder: Nerve strokes are given as a sign of completion of each body part you are massaging. After a while your partner will develop an unspoken understanding that you have just completed massaging a certain body part.

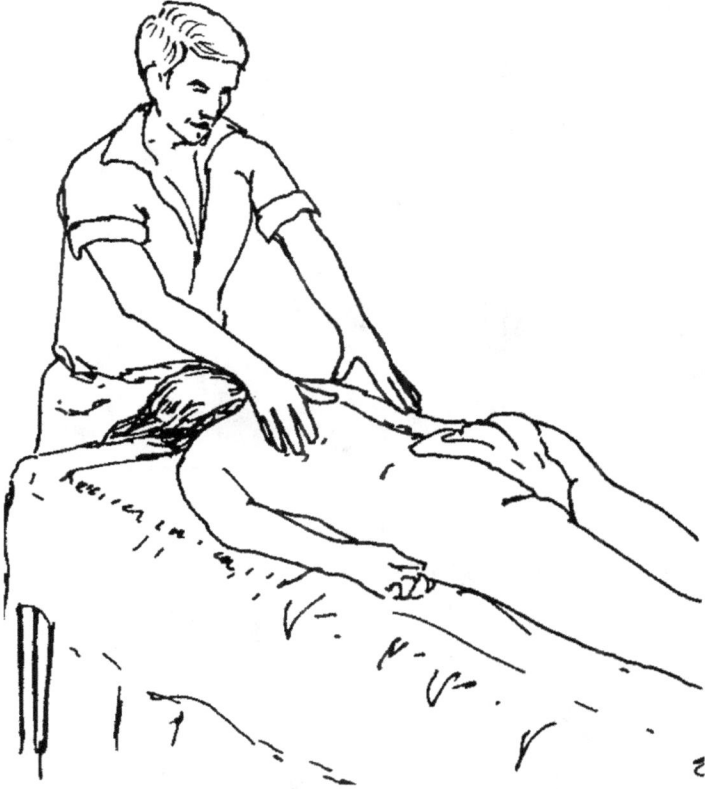

I-74

NERVE STROKES—LET YOUR FINGERS DO THE WALKING, BARELY TOUCHING THE SKIN

WITH YOUR FINGERS. STROKE THE ENTIRE BACK AND THE ARMS AS WELL.

CHAPTER - 4
Finishing Touches

You are almost done. With a soft paper towel, wipe any remaining massage oil off your partner while he or she is still facing down.

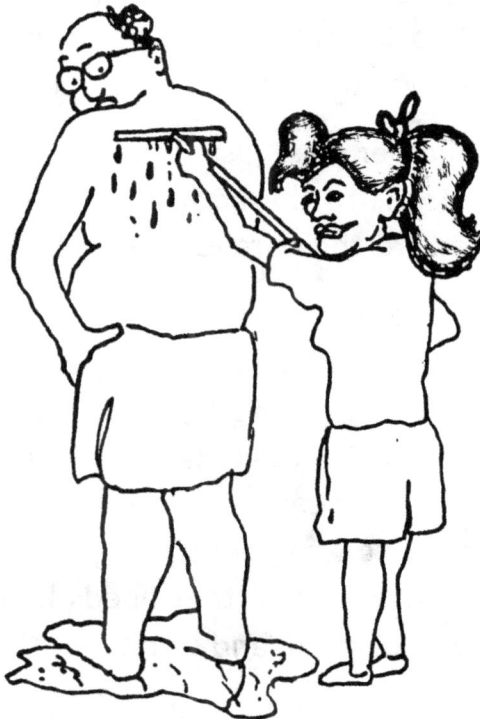

I-75

"STAND UP STRAIGHT AND LET ME FINISH REMOVING THE OIL WITH MY SQUEEGEE."

Communicate a Loving Message

This part has nothing to do with massage but is spiritual in nature, and you may appreciate it. A loving message is the opposite of a selfish act. As a matter of fact, everything you did till now is a giving and nurturing act. Now you will be adding another one.

You have completed this wonderful massage on your partner. Your partner is feeling totally relaxed and wonderful all over. This is a rare moment of tranquility of mind and body connection, not to be missed. The mood is set. This is an excellent time for you to transmit a loving message.

As you remember, we just completed nerve strokes throughout the trunk of the body. Continue with your last nerve strokes toward the ears. Cup your hands gently over your partner's ears.

Picture in your mind a splendid glow of divine light. That light is a giving light. This light represents abundance, goodness of everything in the entire universe, things such as physical health, mental health, prosperity, love, and peace of mind. Think in a loving way about your partner and wish for something you know your partner needs badly. It could be good health, peace of mind, and so on.

See in your mind how all channels are opening. This divine, giving light starts to flow towards you and it enters through your head filling you with a magnificent glow. Try seeing yourself as if you are outside of your own body witnessing this magnificent sight. The light has filled you completely.

You become one with the light—you become the conduit between the splendid light and your partner. The light continues to flow from you to your healing hands and from there to your partner's ears and head as well as to the rest of his body. The light engulfs your partner's body, filling it with its glow and splendor. Visualize how the light is cradling your partner's body in a loving way. As the light continues to flow it starts to exit out from your partner's feet. As this magnificent glow is leaving your partner's body, it removes all impurity from his or her body, leaving behind an abundance of good health, peace of mind, prosperity, love and everything else you wished for.

Visualize your partner receive healing as a result of the light going through him or her. There is no question in your mind that healing has become a reality. For you it is not a "maybe," for you it's an undisputed fact that your partner is one hundred percent healed. Your kind wish for somebody other than yourself has materialized.

A Final Gentle Rocking

- Stand by your partner's side.

- Place one hand on his or her shoulder and the other on your partner's hip and gently rock your partner like a loving mother would rock her baby. This action has a beautiful sedating and peaceful effect.

- Do that for about a minute, then let go.

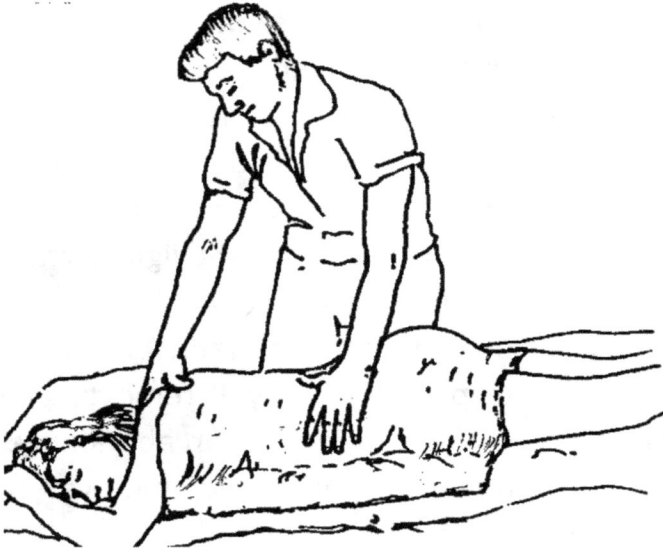

I-76

ROCKING YOUR PARTNER AT THE END OF THE MASSAGE HAS A CALMING, SOOTHING EFFECT.

Now your massage is completed. If your partner fell asleep, that's natural. Just let it be. Allow your partner to wake up naturally. If your partner is awake, ask, "How do you feel?" Most likely, you will receive sincere and grateful compliments such as: "It was absolutely wonderful." "It was great." "I never felt better in my life." Or, as one lady once told me, "I am yet to decide which one is better massage or sex?"

Don't be afraid to ask your partner to swap massages with you. It will not only make you feel good, but by experiencing it, you will be able to improve your technique and become a better massage giver. Keep practicing your technique. Just like everything else, practice makes perfect; you will become good at it and will gain confidence doing it. After a while you will find that you know the strokes and the technique by heart and won't need the book that much.

If you are attentive enough to the person you are massaging, it will be noticed and appreciated. If someone has specific pain, devote more time to the area in which he or she has a problem. Just go to the chapter where the problem is described and spend time relieving the pain. Don't be surprise if your love life improves as a side effect of giving massage. Most likely it's going to bring the two of you closer together, more then ever. Above all, you'll feel terrific whether you are the giver or the receiver. Enjoy.

www.ingramcontent.com/pod-product-compliance
Lightning Source LLC
Chambersburg PA
CBHW050534280326
41933CB00011B/1584